Thuja Occidentalis

MINIMUM SYNDROME OF MAXIMUM VALUE

THUJA OCCIDENTALIS

A REFLECTION FROM THE CLINICAL BEDSIDE

BY

PROF. L.M. KHAN

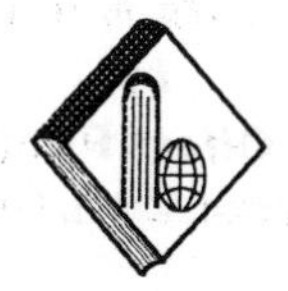

B. JAIN PUBLISHERS (P) LTD.
INDIA

NOTE FROM THE PUBLISHERS

Any information given in this book is not intended to be taken as a replacement for medical advice. Any person with a condition requiring medical attention should consult a qualified practitioner or therapist.

First Edition : 2003

Price: Rs. 20.00

Published by

Kuldeep Jain

for

B. Jain Publishers (P) Ltd.

1921, Chuna Mandi, St. 10th Paharganj,
New Delhi-110 055

Ph: 23580800, 23581100, 23581300, 23583100
Fax: 011-23580471
Website: www.bjainbooks.com, Email: bjain@vsnl.com

PRINTED IN INDIA

by

J.J. Offset Printers

522, FIE, Patpar Ganj, Delhi-110 092

ISBN : 81-8056-366-9
BOOK CODE : BK-5719

CONTENTS

INTRODUCTION

THUJA OCCIDENTALIS

{TREE OF LIFE or ARBOR VITAE}

The cypress was regarded as a SACRED TREE by many people. Thanks to its longevity and evergreen leaves, the cypress – Thuja was called the Tree of life.

The Ancient Greeks and Romans associated it with Underworld deities. It was the tree of the regions below, linked with the worship of Pluto[1] and for this reason, planted in graveyards.

It owed its places as the funeral tree around the whole Mediterranean Basin to the common symbolism of the Conifer, its incorruptible resin and evergreen leaves suggesting immortality and resurrection. 'Winter frosts only emphasis the powers of resistance possessed by the cypress, from which they cannot take its leaves'.

In ancient China it was believed that longevity could be obtained by eating cypress seeds, because they were rich in *yang* substances. To rub the heels with cypress resin enabled one to walk on water, since it makes the body light. Jade and Gold

[1] God of the Underworld.

could be found by the light of burning cypress resin, they being yang substances and symbols of immortality.

The American Arbo vitae is a "spiry evergreen attaining a height of from 20 to 50 feet, though generally not above 40, and a diameter of about 10-20 feet through the greatest breadth of foliage. It abounds in the upper zones of North America, from Pennsylvania northwards, where it often forms what are commonly known as cedar swamps. It grows upon the *rocky banks of rivers*, and in *low, swampy spots*, blossoming from May until June and maturing its fruit in autumn – The Arbo vitae assumes a conical form with such true lines as to appear 'clipped', thus forming one of our most valuable high-hedge trees". (Millspaugh)

Thuja was introduced to France from Canada in the reign of Francis I. of France, and it has now an honoured place in most of our gardens and shrubberies. The native habitat of Thuja is not without its importance in relation to therapeutics. *It loves SWAMPS*.

THUJA OCCIDENTALIS

NOMEN OMEN

{TREE OF LIFE or ARBOR VITAE}

NATURAL ORDER : CONIFERAE

PREPARATION : The green leaves of Thuja occidentalis are first bruised to a fine pulp by themselves then stirred up with two thirds of their weight of alcohol and then the juice is expressed.

HISTORY OF INCLUSION OF THUJA AS AN ANTYSYCOTIC REMEDY

A young clergymen came to Hahnemann complaining of a greenish urethral discharge, pimples on the glans penis & some swelling. He stoutly denied any wrong doing. Hahnemann did not give him any medicine and ask him to report after three days. He returned without any symptom after three days. He then recalled that while sauntering through the garden he had plucked and chewed a spring of arbor vitae. This case led Hahnemann to prove the remedy and all manifestations produced were of sycotic diathesis (personality) including urethral discharge.

Hahnemann says, in Materia Medica Pura, "the juice of Thuja must be specifically useful in those hideous diseases arising from impure coitus – the figwarts, if they are not complicated with other miasmata, and the experience also shows that *Thuja is only efficacious remedy for them.* It also cures the bad kind of Gonorrhoea resulting from impure coitus if it is not complicated with other miasmata". Hahnemann used 30th potency earlier then he found 60th potency (Vigesillion Fold) more useful.

This antisycotic remedy corrects certain states of the system thus remaining the obstruction in the curative action of the other, seemingly, indicated remedies. Thuja, for instance, cures or so changes the existing conditions that other remedies cure which did not do so before Thuja was given. For example, a case of enuresis had resisted many seemingly indicated remedies until the hands were discovered to be covered with warts, when a few drops of Thuja cured.

THUJA OCCIDENTALIS has the power to produce most important pathogenesis in the *mucous membrane of genito-urinary system and intestine, and skin.*

On mind, it produces many types of symptomatology starting from fixed ideas to different feelings like sadness, ill humor, etc. Thuja also has affinity for *glands, ovaries, nerves, occiput and left sided affections.*

It is the medicine capable of producing great prostration, rapid emaciation and soft exuberant, fungoid lesions – warts, condylomata, polypi, especially pedunculated (with a narrow stalk; Latin *pedis* 'the foot'), blackish in appearance or suppressed, etc.

Thuja has the *specific properties* to eradicate the primary stage of sycosis and prevent further complication. In sycotic cases – figwarts, condolymata and wart like excrescences upon the mucus and cutaneous surfaces. *Sulphur* is the specific medicine for primary stages of Psora where the symptoms are on the surface and *Mercury* has got the same relation to syphilis.

NOTE : The curative power of Thuja is confined not only to sycosis but can, like other remedies, cure when the symptoms are indicated and where no sycotic element in the case is apparent.

GONORRHOEA

INTRODUCTION

Many believe that the description of 'an issue of seed' (in flow of seed) in the fifteenth chapter of the book of *Leviticus in the old Testament*, and of the precautions that were to be taken to deal with it, is a reference to this disease.

The causative organism of gonorrhoea – *Neisseria gonorrhoeae*, was discovered by Neisser in 1879 and the complete result of his investigations were published in 1882. Leistikow in 1882 and Buman in 1885 grew the organism on a culture medium and the latter successfully inoculated the male urethra, producing characteristic symptoms and signs of gonorrhoea. The gonococcal compliment fixation test (GFT) was introduced by Muller and Openheim in 1906.

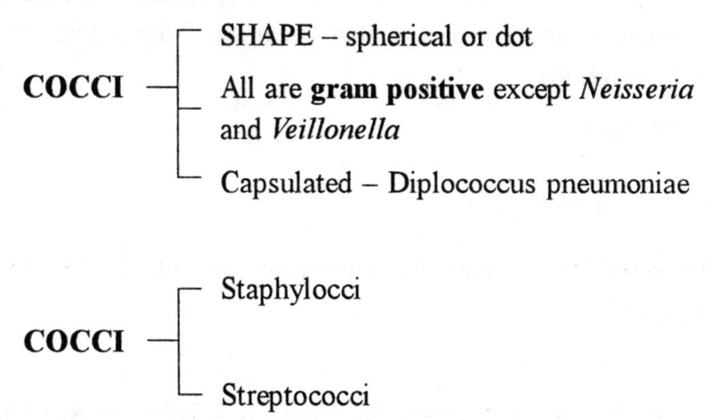

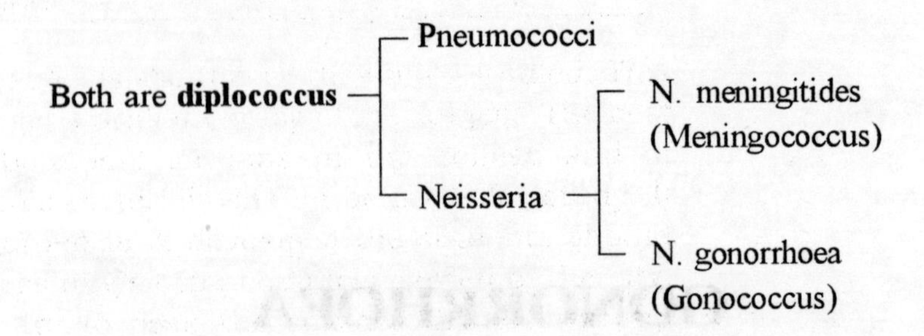

NOTE : Gonococci from the primary isolation of clinical material.

⇩

Typical small colonies develop containing piliated (hair like structure developing from bacterial cell surface) cocci.

ANALOGY – Excess hairy growth on a mole or wart or a single hair on a mole or wart.

COMPARATIVE CLINICAL EVALUATION FOR GONORRHOEA IN MALE AND FEMALE

Clinical diseases are less severe in females, many of whom may carry gonococci in the cervix without developing any clinical symptoms.

WHY? As because the vaginal mucosa is not usually affected in adults, because the stratified squamous epithelium is resistant to infection by the cocci and also because of the acidic ph of vaginal secretions.

Gonorrhoea :

Acquired
Inherited

Acquired gonorrhoea : History of impure coition → primary manifestation – Figwarts.

– Condylomata.

– According to Hahnemann, Thuja is specific, even if it is

applied externally (Q), [the only exception to the external application].

- If primary manifestation is suppressed or cauterized, they return in the same spot or appear in other parts as same or as growth and excresences.

So presence of growth or excrescences suggest the use of Thuja, as Thuja has produced growth like excrescences on its administration and it shows these sycotic taints which may be acquired or inherited. It can be used externally in the old cases of larger excrescences (Hahanemann says), along with internal administration in infinetisimal infrequent doses.

Example of growth or excrescences –

Skin	– Warty excrescences.
	– Condylomata.
	– Epithelioma.
	– Nevus.
Mucous membrane	– Polypi.
	– Moist mucous tubercles.
	– Cauliflower excrescences of os uteri.
	– Nevus.
Blood vessel	– Nrvus.
	– Bleeding fungus growth.
	– Fatty tumors.
	– Excessive venosity.

Inherited gonorrhoea : Parents sycotic taint transmitted to the next offspring. So offsprings are –

- apt to be thin, pale & pot bellied;
- subject to tinea ciliaris;
- prone to caries at the roots of teeth.

- Watery stools that are expelled forcibly with much noisy flatus every day after the break fast.
- Waken from sleep, screaming and confused (*Lycopodium*).

In their early years, they have tendency for warts, scaly eruptions or humid asthma.

DEVELOPMENT OF SYCOSIS

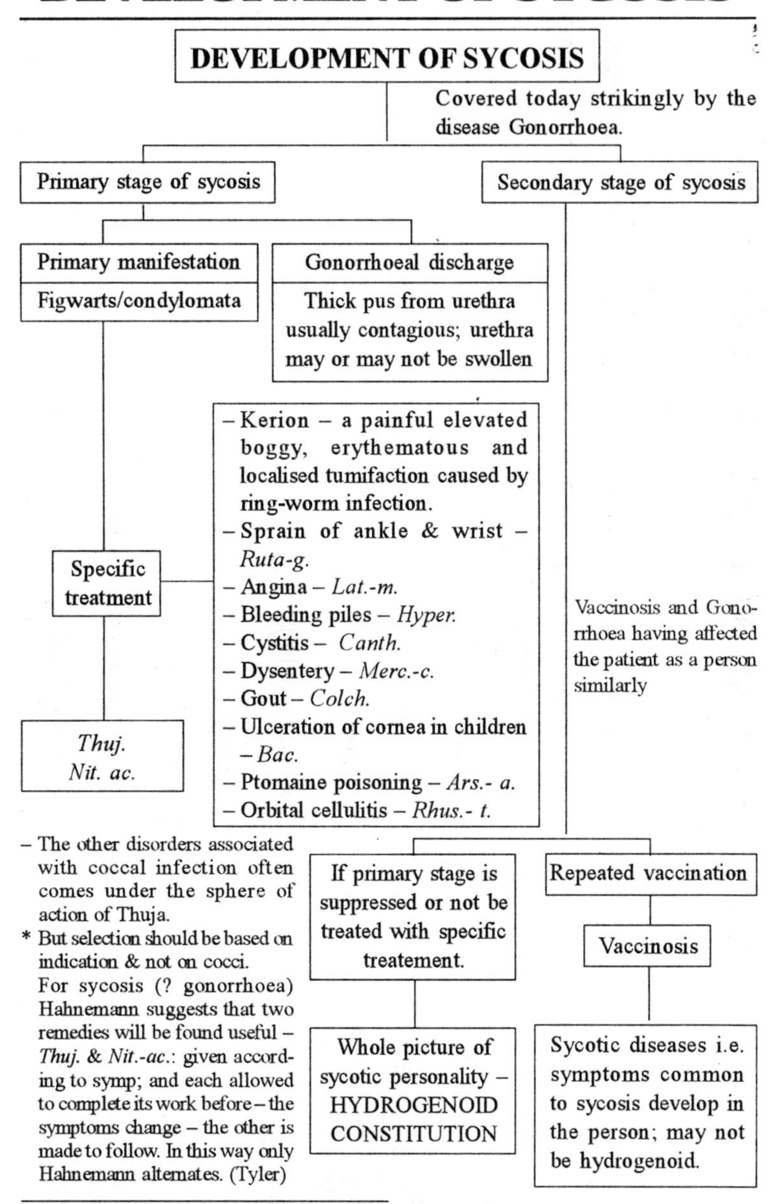

– The other disorders associated with coccal infection often comes under the sphere of action of Thuja.

* But selection should be based on indication & not on cocci.
For sycosis (? gonorrhoea) Hahnemann suggests that two remedies will be found useful – *Thuj.* & *Nit.-ac.*: given according to symp; and each allowed to complete its work before – the symptoms change – the other is made to follow. In this way only Hahnemann alternates. (Tyler)

---

* **Homoeopathy is more interested at bedside & body reaction of patient as a person rather than extrinsic invaders & mankind (e.g. bacteria) – LMK.**

COMPLICATIONS AFTER VACCINATION

Vaccination

Toxic complication Similar to Thuja Pathogenesy

- Inveterate neuralgias.
  - Boring in a small spot in the cheek bones spreading to the head & neck.
  - Violent pressing pain as of a nail being forced into the vertex or the left frontal eminence.
- Eruptions.
- Warty growths.
- Convulsions.
- Rheumatoid arthritis.
- Endocarditis.
- Asthma.
- Depression of immune systum.
- Auto immune diseases, etc.

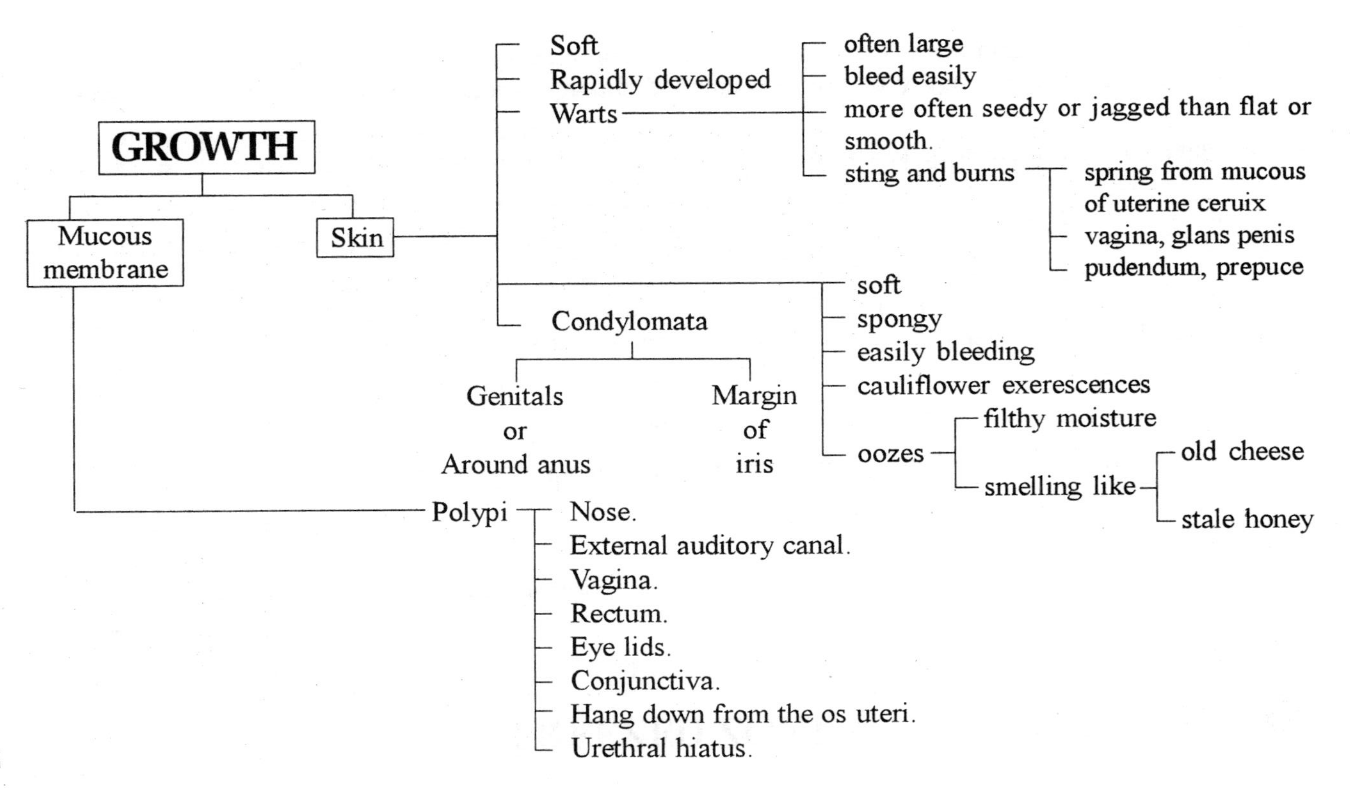
GROWTH
Mucous membrane
Skin
Soft
Rapidly developed
Warts
often large
bleed easily
more often seedy or jagged than flat or smooth.
sting and burns
spring from mucous of uterine ceruix
vagina, glans penis
pudendum, prepuce
Condylomata
soft
spongy
easily bleeding
cauliflower exerescences
oozes
filthy moisture
smelling like
old cheese
stale honey
Genitals or Around anus
Margin of iris
Polypi
Nose.
External auditory canal.
Vagina.
Rectum.
Eye lids.
Conjunctiva.
Hang down from the os uteri.
Urethral hiatus.

FREEZED ZONE

|

Looking Sickly

- Scope of Thuja.

1. Person who is much vaccinated.
2. Person who has been excessively sensitive to vaccination.
3. Person who failed to take – react acutely.
4. Person who did not take vaccnation.

Thuja is AN ANTIDOTE TO VACCINATION in its early, acute stage.

- It is a pre-eminently strong madicine for cases where you have the history of snake-bite, small-pox and vaccination.
- A disease state or polluted constitution which is due to vaccinial poison. It has got long lasting polluted constitutional state. The person who suffered from vaccinosis may not be ill or sick in ordinary sense but he must be in a subdued morbid state, he has been blighted.
- The most worse cases of vaccinosis where vaccination did not take place.
- Taking – is the constitutional reaction of a patient as a person & is a good sign.
- In a case of "no taking" the poisonous material has been absorbed in the whole constitution, now taking place gradually in a chronic process with the host of disease syndrome.
- Brnett's vaccinosis – a state of indefnite, chronic, polluted constitution & their manifestation develop in a different form in different personality profile according to their own susceptibility & family & personal predispostion.

FREEZED ZONE *(Contd.)*

FREEZED ZONE

- Gonorrhoea
  - Maltreated
  - Suppressed
  - Chordee*[1]
- Syphilis
- Rheumatism
- Producing inflammation
  - Swelling
  - Ulceration
  - Thick, yellow or greenish muco-pus
- Vaccination — Bad effects of vaccination (*Ant.-c.*, *Sil.*)
- *Epulis (Fibromata)
- *Polyp*[2]
  - Foul
  - Moist
  - Nasal
  - Rectal, etc.
- *Naevi
- Papillomata*[3]

* Due to chronic irritation by discharges, Thuja will change this poisonous discharge; that may cause the growths to dwindle (but slowly), it often does something after their removal to prevent relapse.

1. painful inflammatory downward curving of penis.
2. an innocent stalked tumor of surface/lining epithelium.
3. papillomatosis – the condition of being affected & papillomata.
   papillomatous – having the characteristics of relating to papilloma.

FREEZED ZONE *(Contd.)*

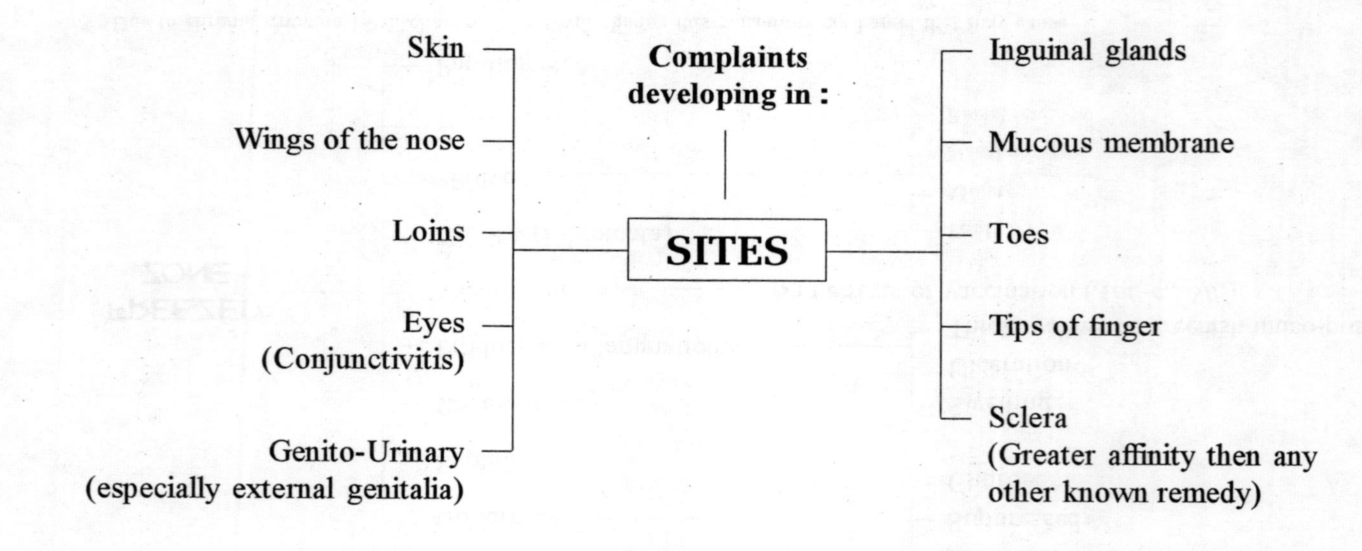

FREEZED ZONE *(Contd.)*

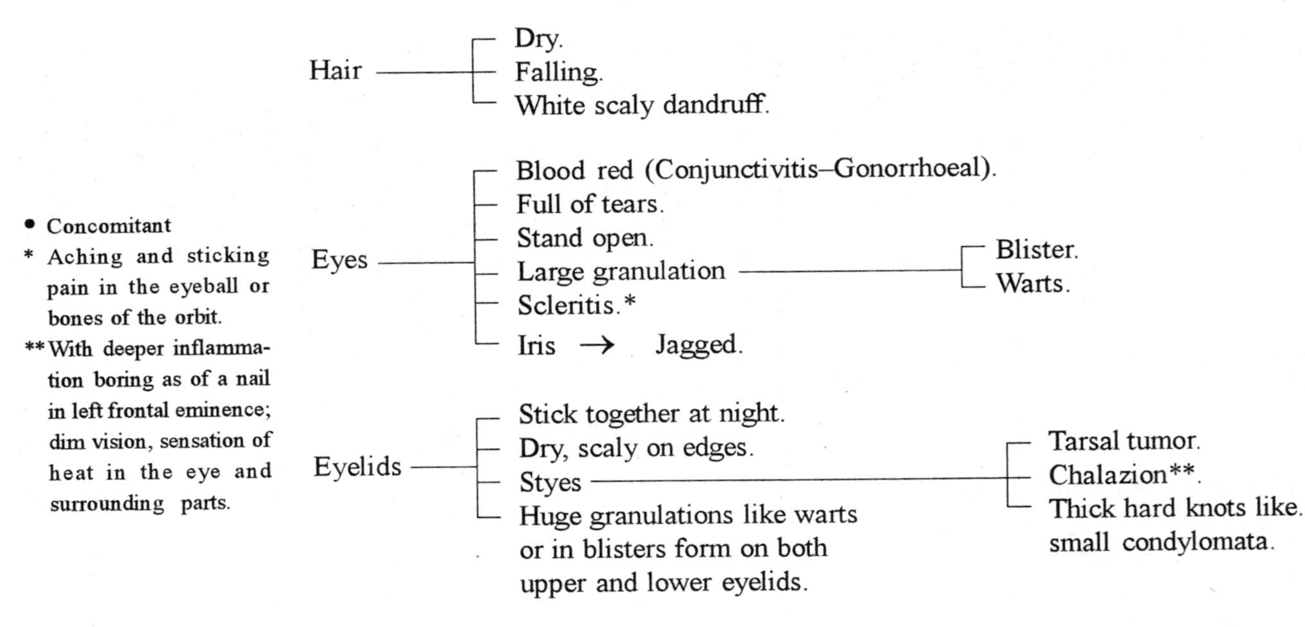

- Concomitant

* Aching and sticking pain in the eyeball or bones of the orbit.

** With deeper inflammation boring as of a nail in left frontal eminence; dim vision, sensation of heat in the eye and surrounding parts.

* Inflammation of the sclera.

** Small eyelid mass due to inflammation of a meibomian gland.

FREEZED ZONE *(Contd.)*

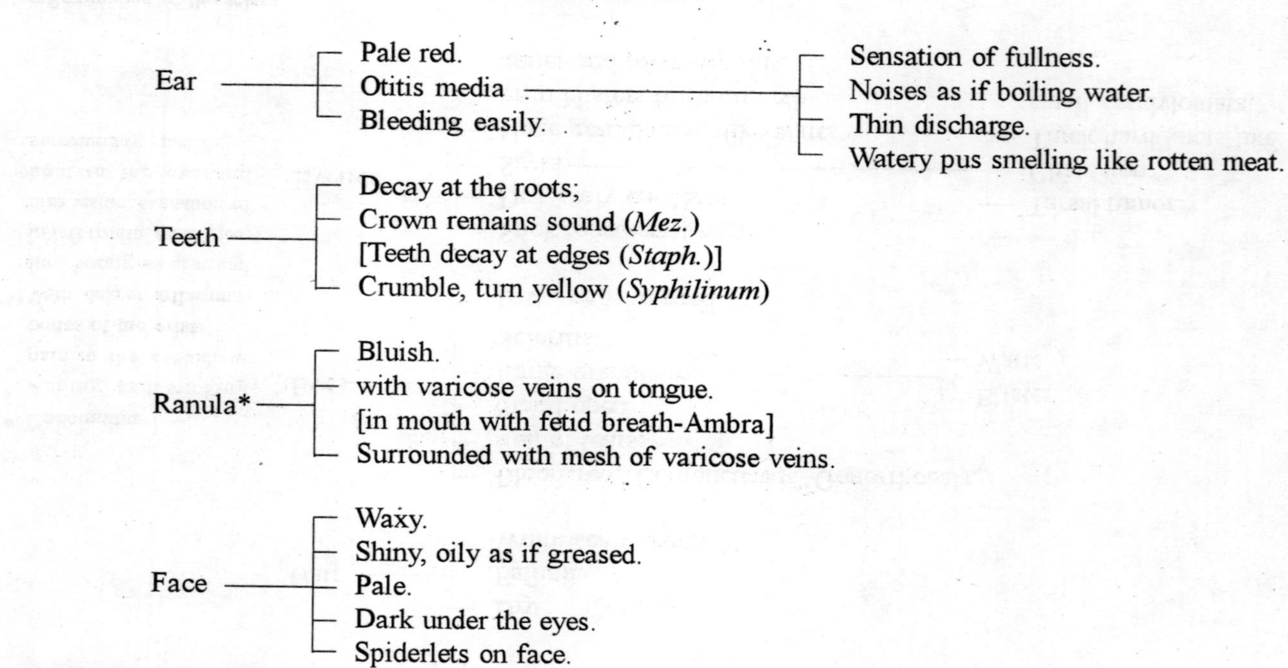

* A cystic tumor beneath the tongue.

FREEZED ZONE *(Contd.)*

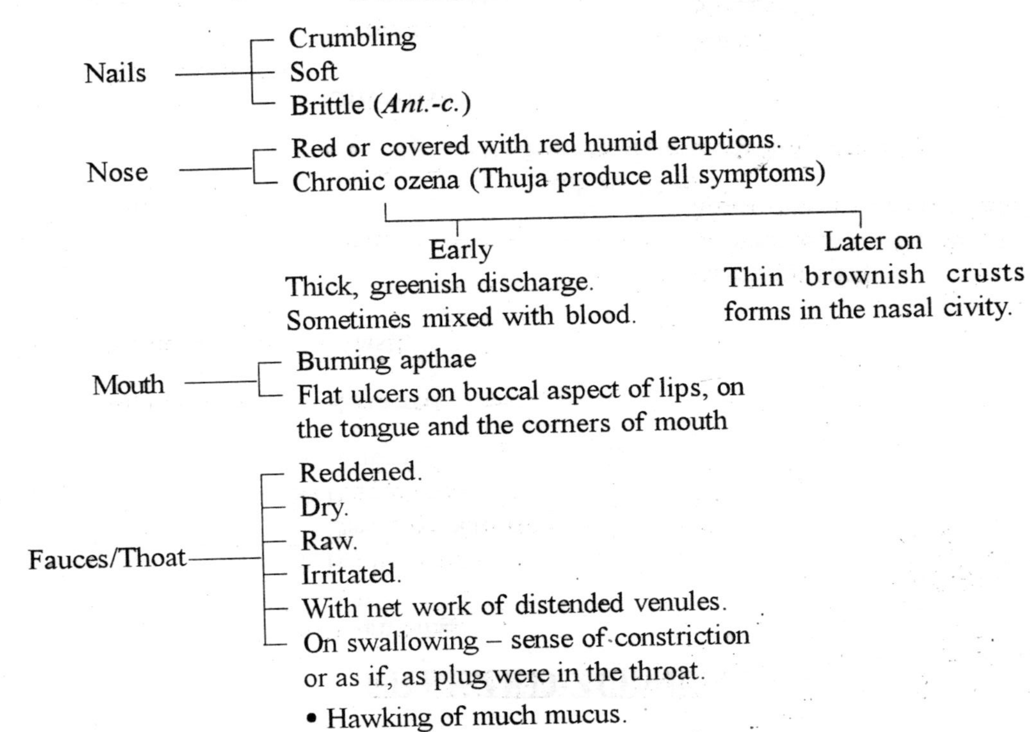

FREEZED ZONE *(Contd.)*

- Nails
  - Crumbling
  - Soft
  - Brittle (*Ant.-c.*)
  - Distored, deformed
  - Discolored
  - Ribbed
- Nipples — Retracted
- Perineum — Moist
- Anus
  - Fissure
    - Painful to touch
    - Surrounded with flat warts
    - Moist mucous condylomata*
  - Piles
    - Swollen, Painful
    - Pain more severe while sitting
- Male Genitalia
  - Offensive
  - Prepuce
    - Puffed
    - Sloughy**

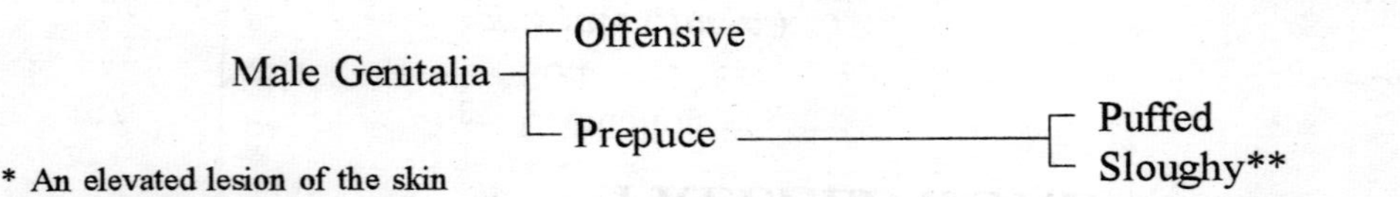
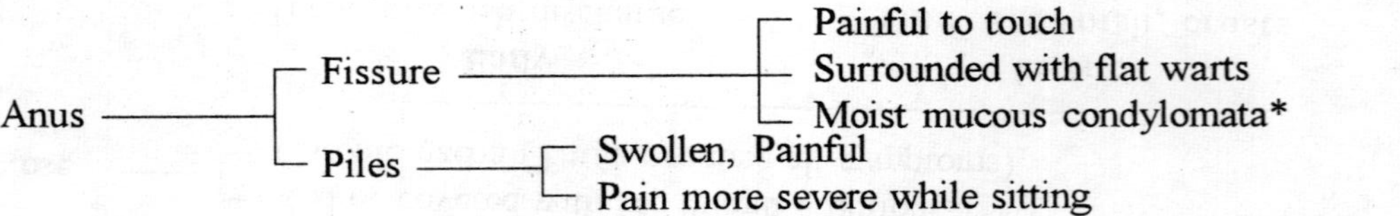
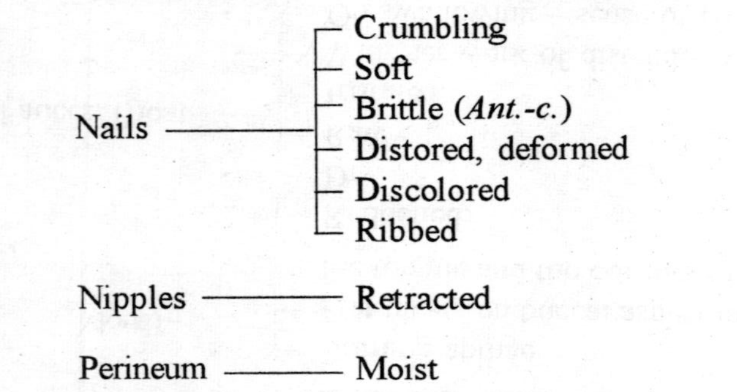

* An elevated lesion of the skin

** Dead tissue; giving of cast.

FREEZED ZONE *(Concld.)*

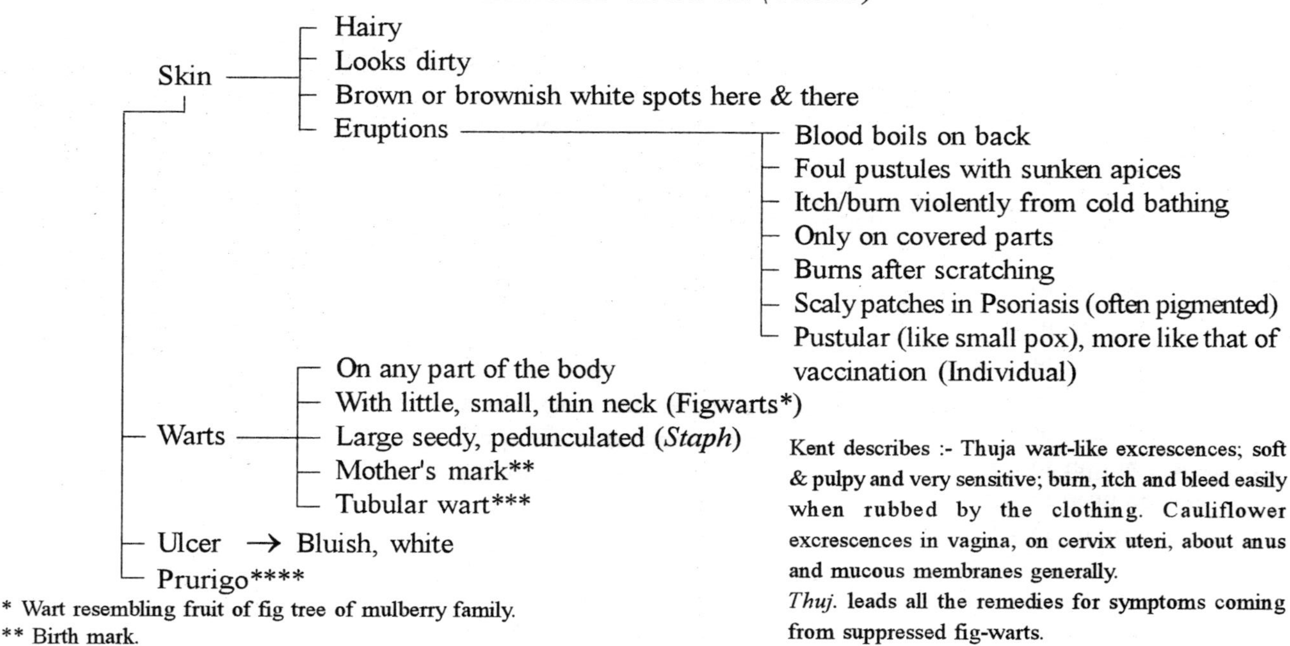

Kent describes :- Thuja wart-like excrescences; soft & pulpy and very sensitive; burn, itch and bleed easily when rubbed by the clothing. Cauliflower excrescences in vagina, on cervix uteri, about anus and mucous membranes generally.

Thuj. leads all the remedies for symptoms coming from suppressed fig-warts.

* Wart resembling fruit of fig tree of mulberry family.

** Birth mark.

*** Long wart, the same size all the way out.

**** Any of the several itchy skin eruptions in which the characteristic lesion is dome shaped with a small transient vesicle on top.

PATIENT AS A PERSON

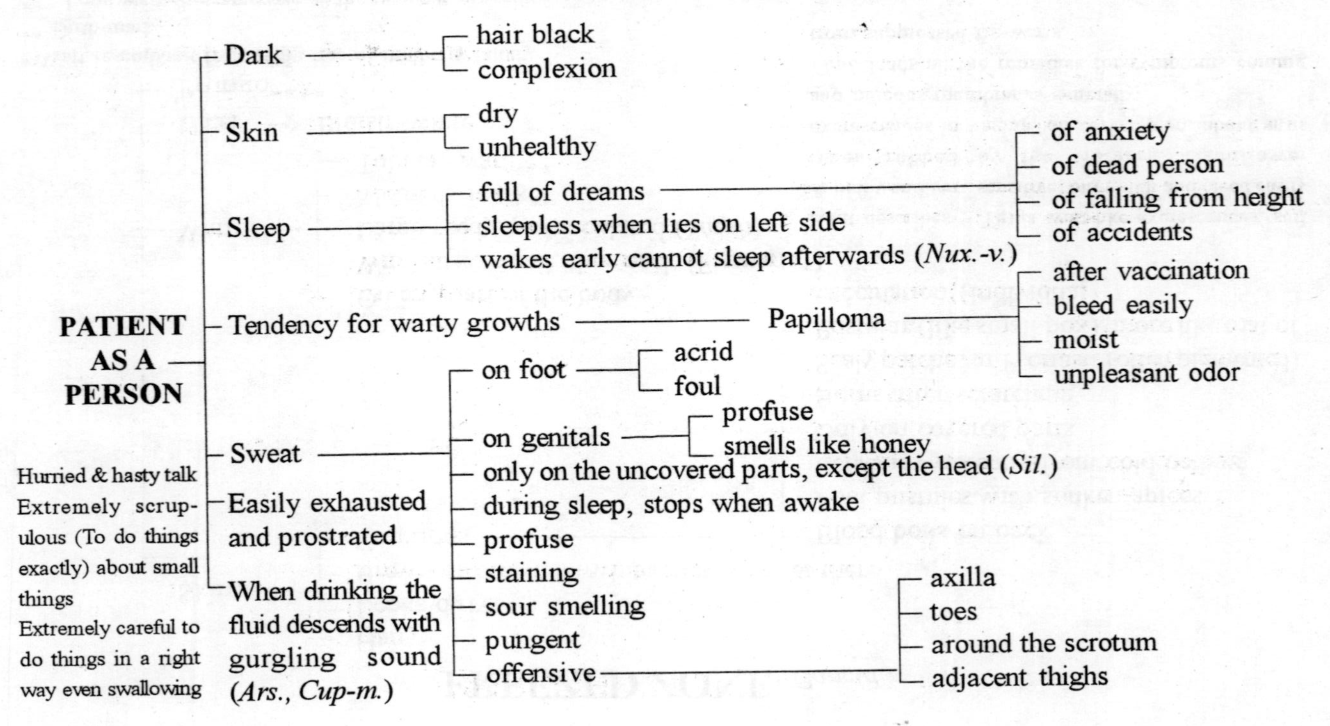

PATIENT AS A PERSON *(Contd.)*

Personality Profile

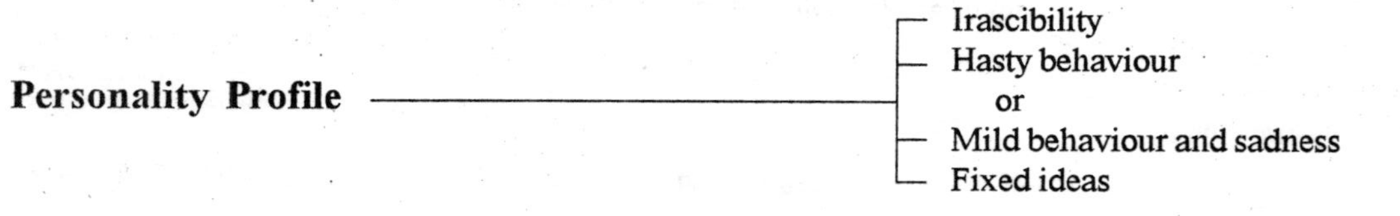

- Irascibility
- Hasty behaviour
- or
- Mild behaviour and sadness
- Fixed ideas

- Exuberant proliferation of epithelial tissues.
- Affections of mucous membrane specially genito urinary tract.
- Discharges – offensive.
- Sweat – in localized area
  - sweetish.
  - offensive.

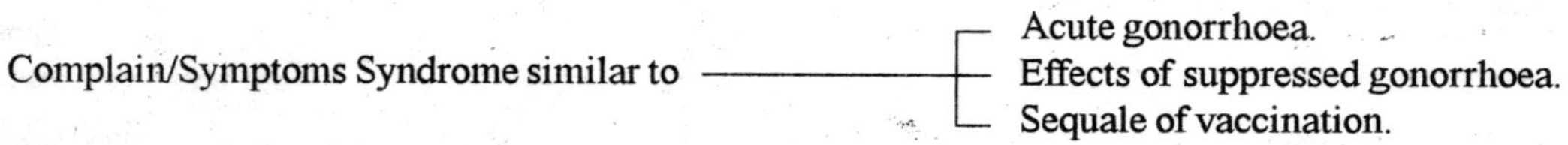

- Complain/Symptoms Syndrome similar to
  - Acute gonorrhoea.
  - Effects of suppressed gonorrhoea.
  - Sequale of vaccination.
- Worse warmth & cold wet weather.
- Better cold and touching the painful parts.

PATIENT AS A PERSON *(Contd.)*

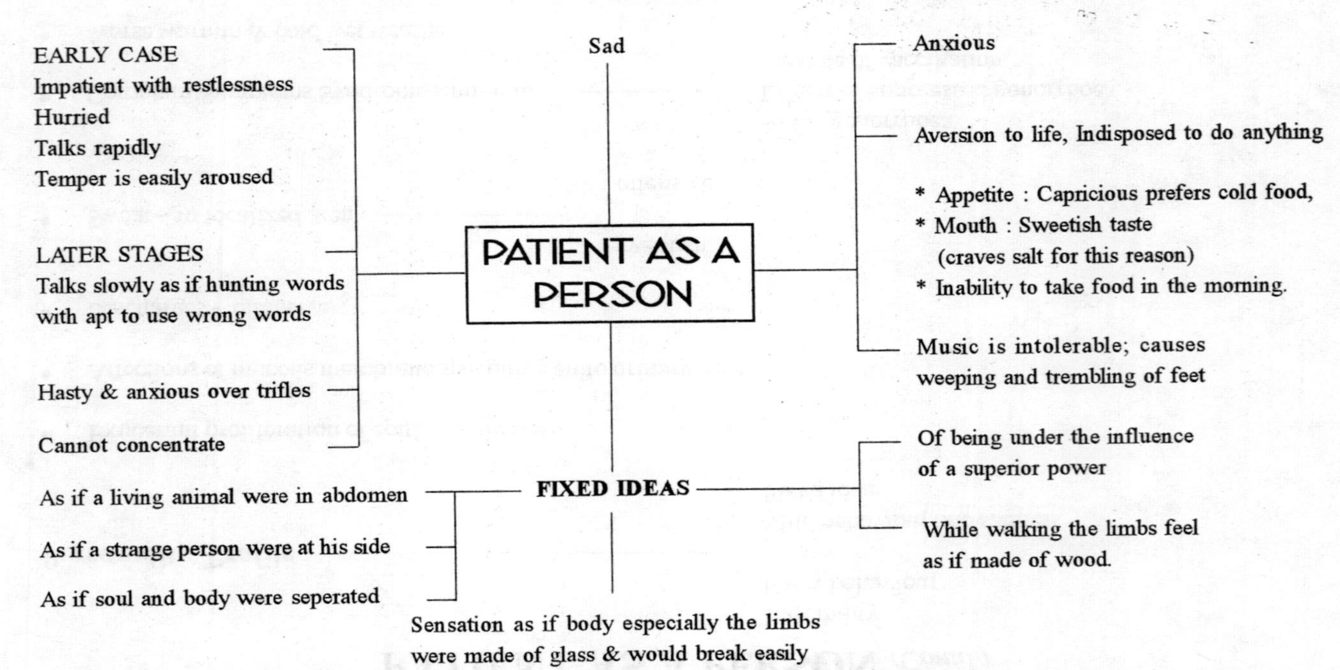

* Very susceptible to gonorrhoeal infection with some other organic poison specially cow pox vaccine.

PATIENT AS A PERSON *(Contd.)*

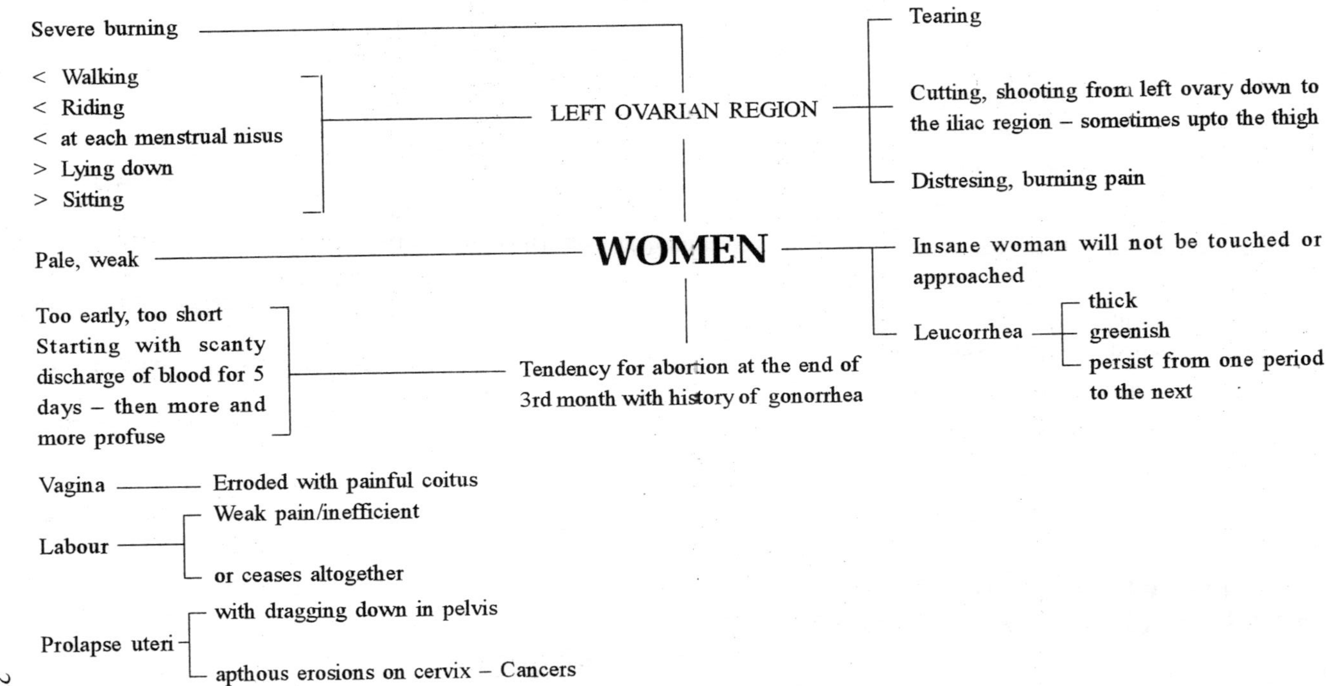

WOMEN *(Contd.)*

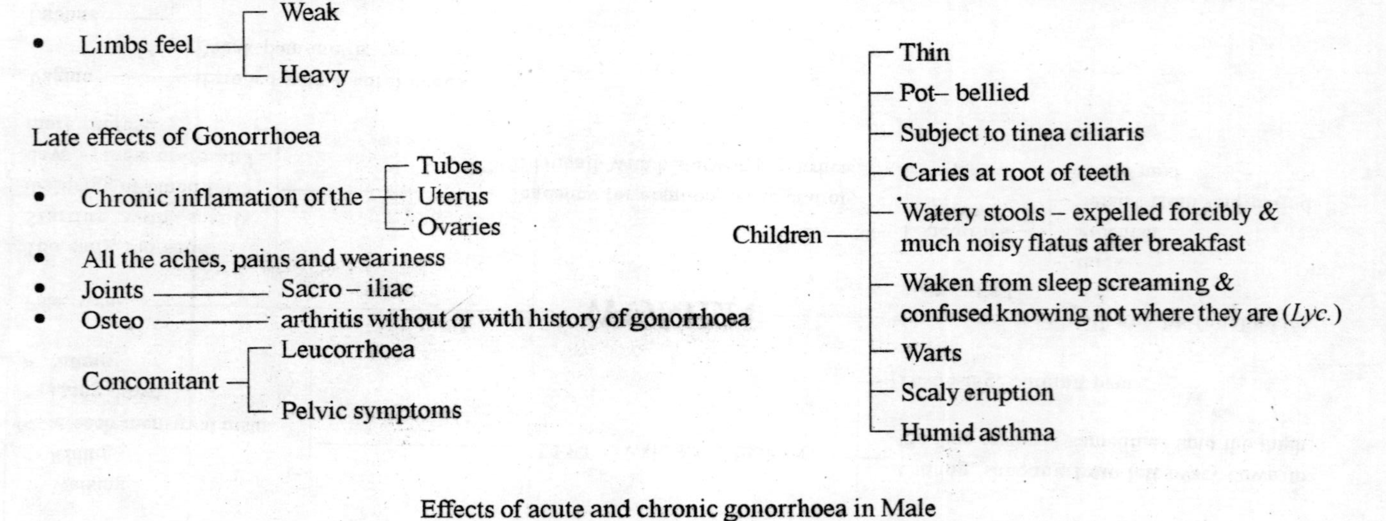

Concomitant :

- Severe pain around left ovary
- Limbs feel — Weak / Heavy

Late effects of Gonorrhoea

- Chronic inflamation of the — Tubes / Uterus / Ovaries
- All the aches, pains and weariness
- Joints — Sacro – iliac
- Osteo — arthritis without or with history of gonorrhoea

Concomitant — Leucorrhoea / Pelvic symptoms

SYCOTIC CONSTITUTION IN SECOND GENERATION

Children —
- Thin
- Pot– bellied
- Subject to tinea ciliaris
- Caries at root of teeth
- Watery stools – expelled forcibly & much noisy flatus after breakfast
- Waken from sleep screaming & confused knowing not where they are (*Lyc.*)
- Warts
- Scaly eruption
- Humid asthma

Effects of acute and chronic gonorrhoea in Male

- Urethritis
- Balanitis
- Prostatitis
- Varicocele
- Ulcers
- Condylomata

MEDICINE AS A REMEDY

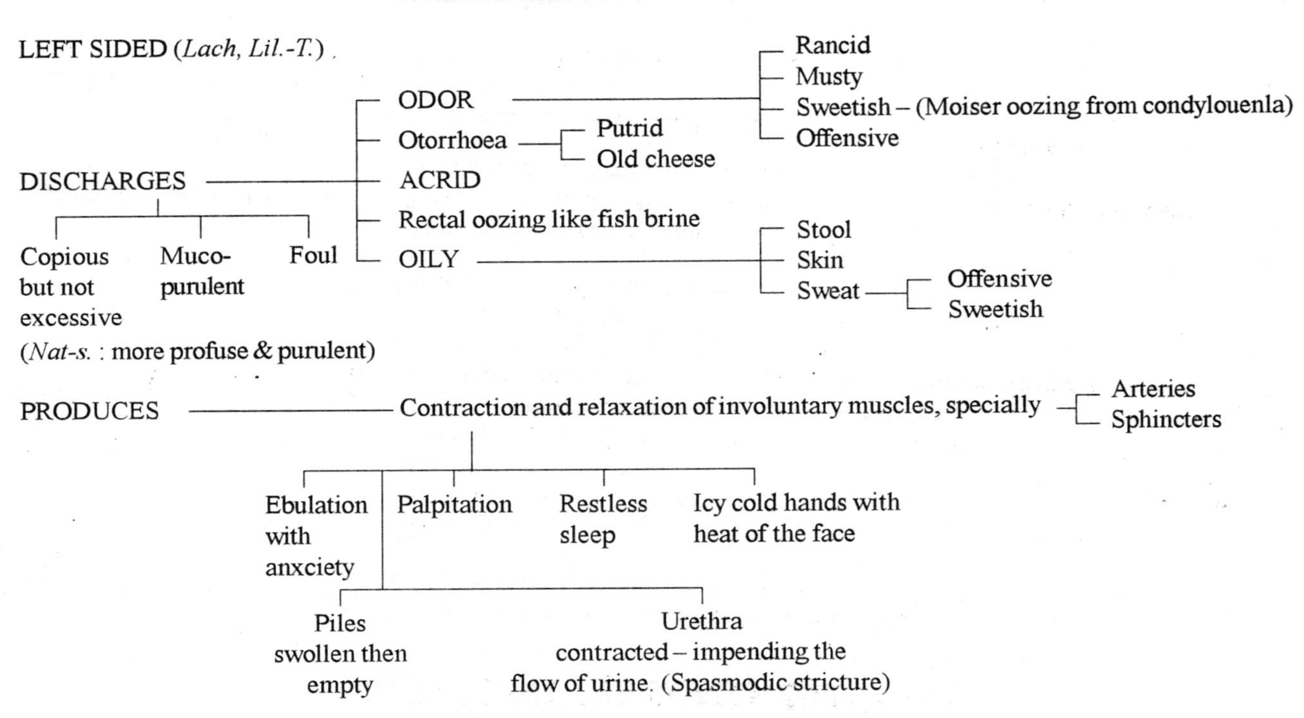

MEDICINE AS A REMEDY *(Contd.)*

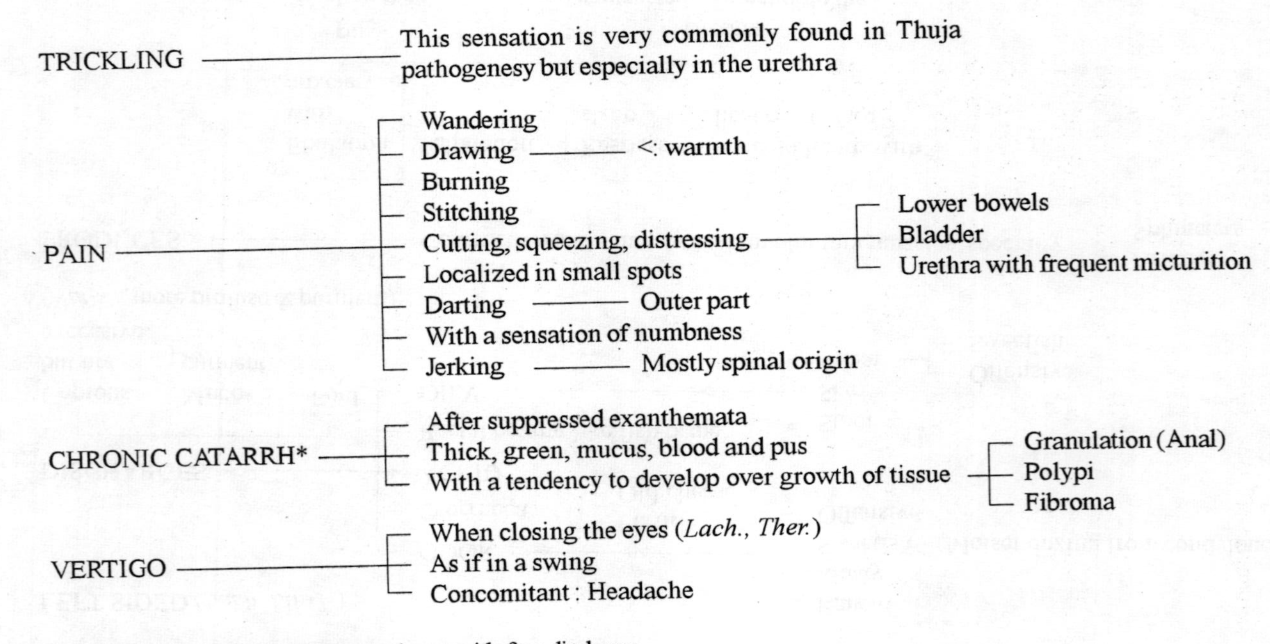

* Inflammation of the mucous membrane with free discharge.

MEDICINE AS A REMEDY *(Contd.)*

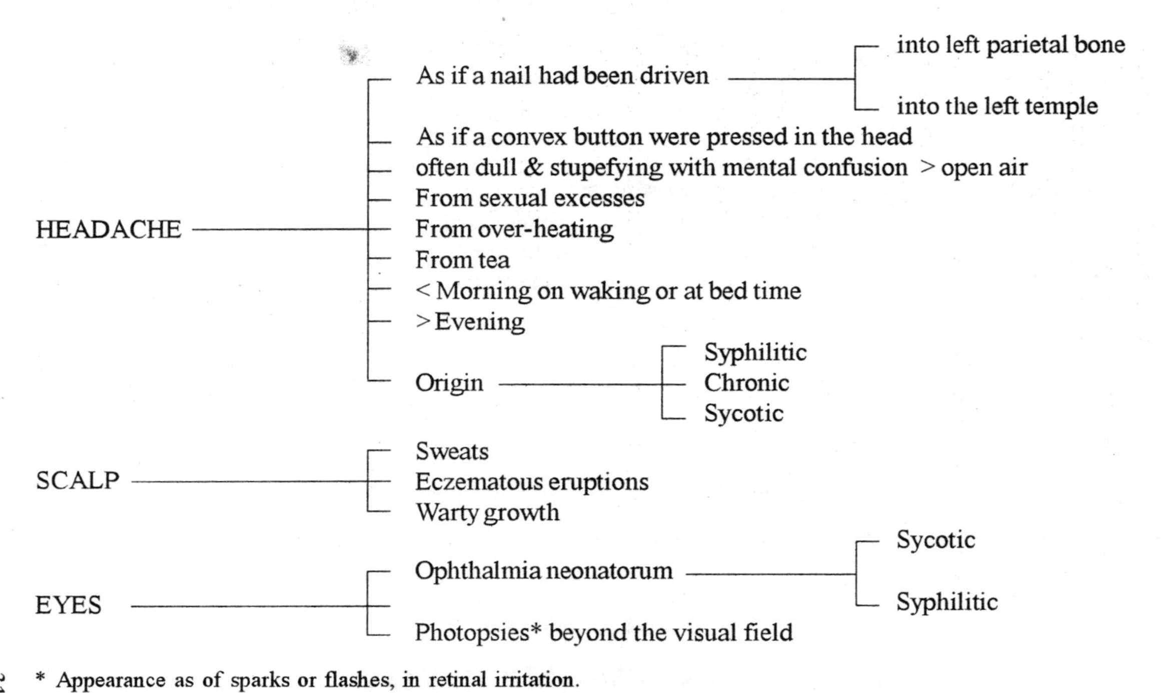

* Appearance as of sparks or flashes, in retinal irritation.

MEDICINE AS A REMEDY *(Contd.)*

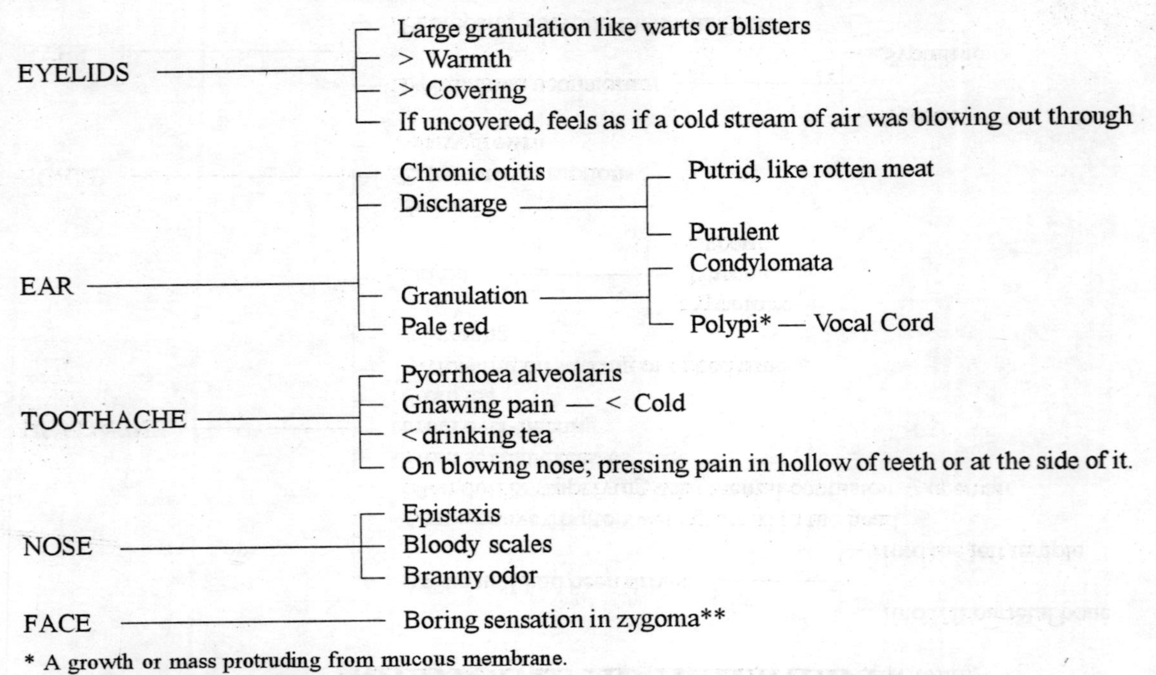

* A growth or mass protruding from mucous membrane.

** Zygomatic process of temporal bone of skull.

MEDICINE AS A REMEDY *(Contd.)*

ERUCTATION
- Rancid
- Noisy

TEETH
- Caries in the root
- Crown sound

GUMS
- Swollen
- Inflammed

MOUTH
- Ranula
- Epulis

TONGUE
- Clean or thinly coated
- Often red and painful
  (Tea drinkers tongue)

- Chronic Pharyngitis with swollen veins

ASTHMA WITH GENERAL SYMPTOMS
- < damp cold
- <: 3 a.m., 3 p.m.
- History of gonorrhoea
- History of repeated vaccination
- Tea drinking

- Arsenic album is acute

MEDICINE AS A REMEDY *(Contd.)*

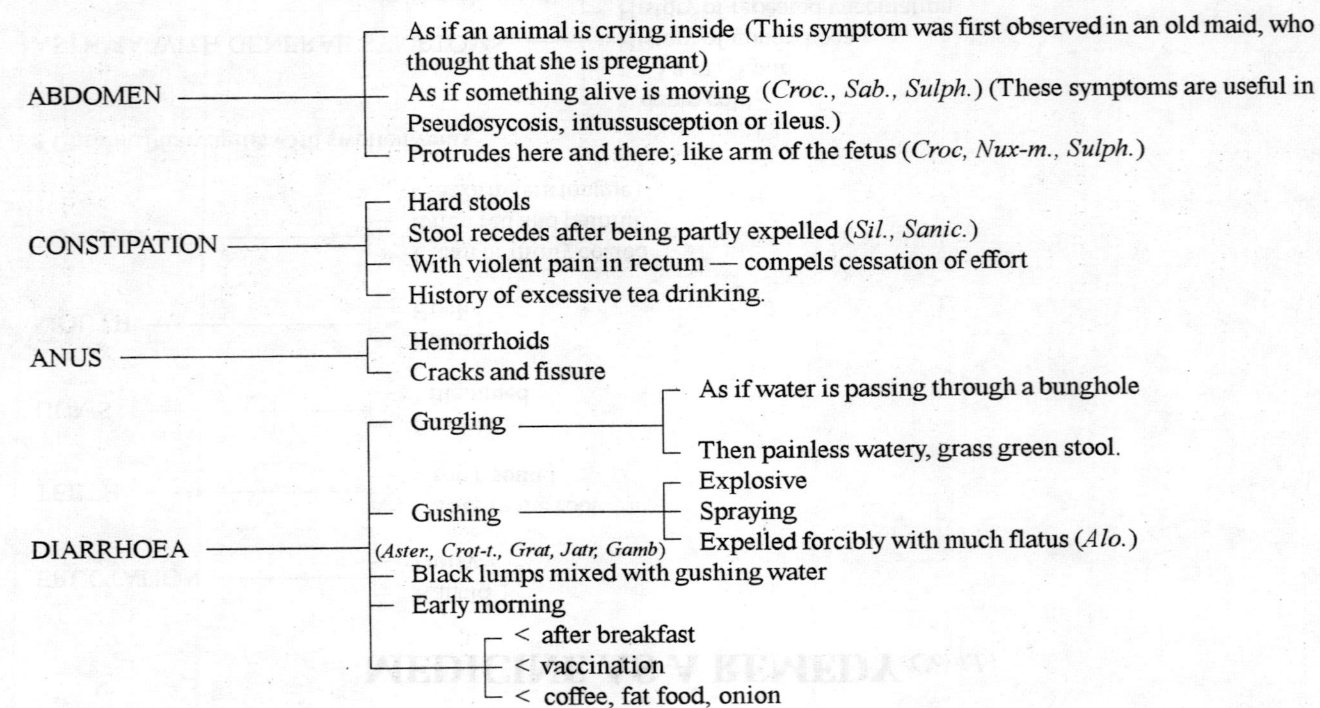

- ABDOMEN
  - As if an animal is crying inside (This symptom was first observed in an old maid, who thought that she is pregnant)
  - As if something alive is moving (*Croc.*, *Sab.*, *Sulph.*) (These symptoms are useful in Pseudosycosis, intussusception or ileus.)
  - Protrudes here and there; like arm of the fetus (*Croc*, *Nux-m.*, *Sulph.*)
- CONSTIPATION
  - Hard stools
  - Stool recedes after being partly expelled (*Sil.*, *Sanic.*)
  - With violent pain in rectum — compels cessation of effort
  - History of excessive tea drinking.
- ANUS
  - Hemorrhoids
  - Cracks and fissure
- DIARRHOEA
  - Gurgling
    - As if water is passing through a bunghole
    - Then painless watery, grass green stool.
  - Gushing
    - Explosive
    - Spraying
    - Expelled forcibly with much flatus (*Alo.*)
  - (*Aster.*, *Crot-t.*, *Grat*, *Jatr*, *Gamb*)
  - Black lumps mixed with gushing water
  - Early morning
  - < after breakfast
  - < vaccination
  - < coffee, fat food, onion

MEDICINE AS A REMEDY *(Contd.)*

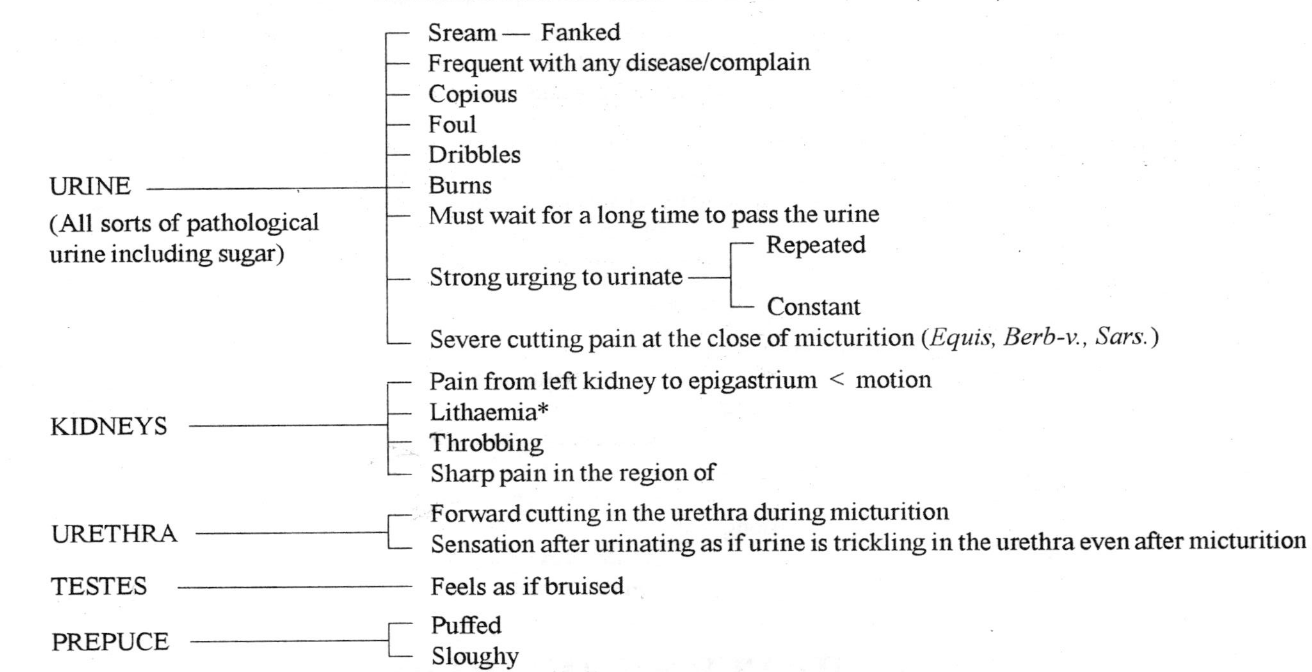

* Condition marked by formation of calculi and concretions.

MEDICINE AS A REMEDY *(Contd.)*

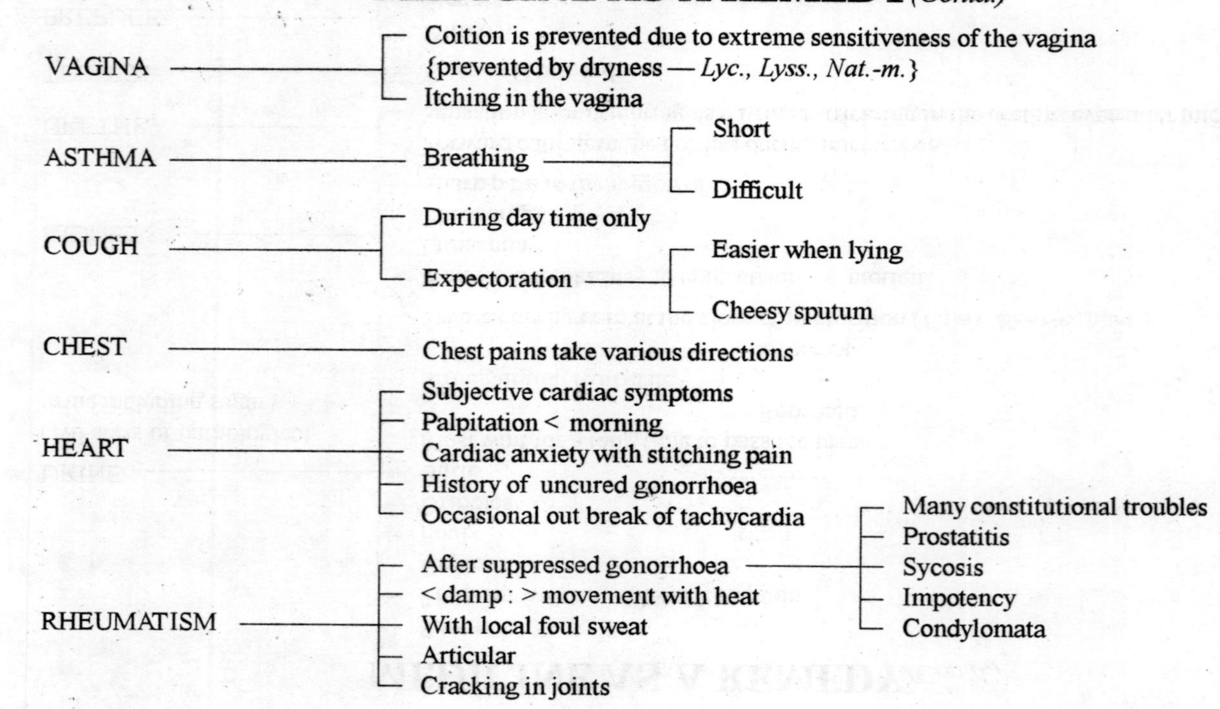

MEDICINE AS A REMEDY *(Contd.)*

ARTHRITIS — Wtih history of Pyorrhoea

BACK — Atrophy of long muscles, severe backache (similar to the small pox symptom)

EXTREMITIES — Limbs feel paralysed

***Myositis ossificans** — Formation of bony masses in muscles, tendons, fascia, aponeurosis, ligaments &bones. Prescribed on general symptoms.

HIPS — Gives way

KNEES — Restless

FINGERS —
- Numb on waking at night (*Nat-m.*)
- Crawling or inflamed fingers or tips of toes

SOLES — Painful

CHILL —
- 3 a.m. and 3 p.m.
- Begins in thighs
- Shaking with yawning
- < during micturition
- Not relieved by heat

HEAT —
- Rises into chest
- With icy cold hands
- With nose bleed or cough

* (Myositis) — Inflammation of voluntary muscles.

PRIME INDICATION

Warty and fungoid growths/styes & tarsal tumors.

Sweat
- Uncovered parts.
- During sleep.
- Sweetish on genitals.

Pain in small spots

Discharges
- Thin
  - Watery, greenish from male urethra with dysuria.
  - Sensation as if drops of urine are trickling down the urethra after mucturition.
- Thick — Greenish leucorrhoea.

Sensation
- as of a plug in throat.
- of something alive in abdomen.

Epidemic of small pox
- Prenentive.
- Curative.

Pre-eminent remedy for any illness following
- Mal treated gonorrhoea.
- Vaccination.
- History of snake bite — animal poisoing.
- History of Small pox.

Thuj. aborts the disease, prevents the pitting when the disease has developed.

GENERAL MODALITIES

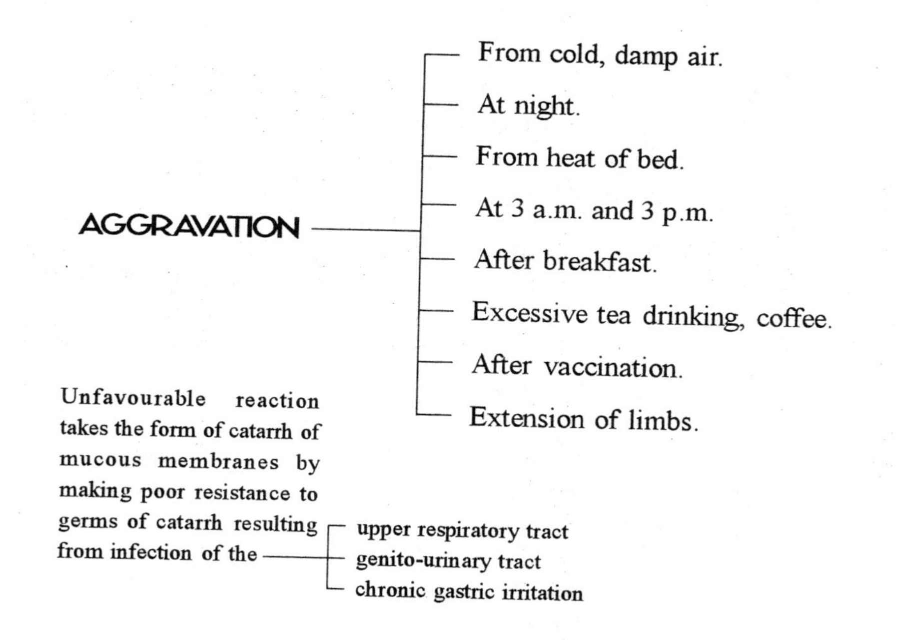

- Clarke said that people who are vaccinated & drink tea; Thuja is best suited to them.

GENERAL MODALITIES *(Concld.)*

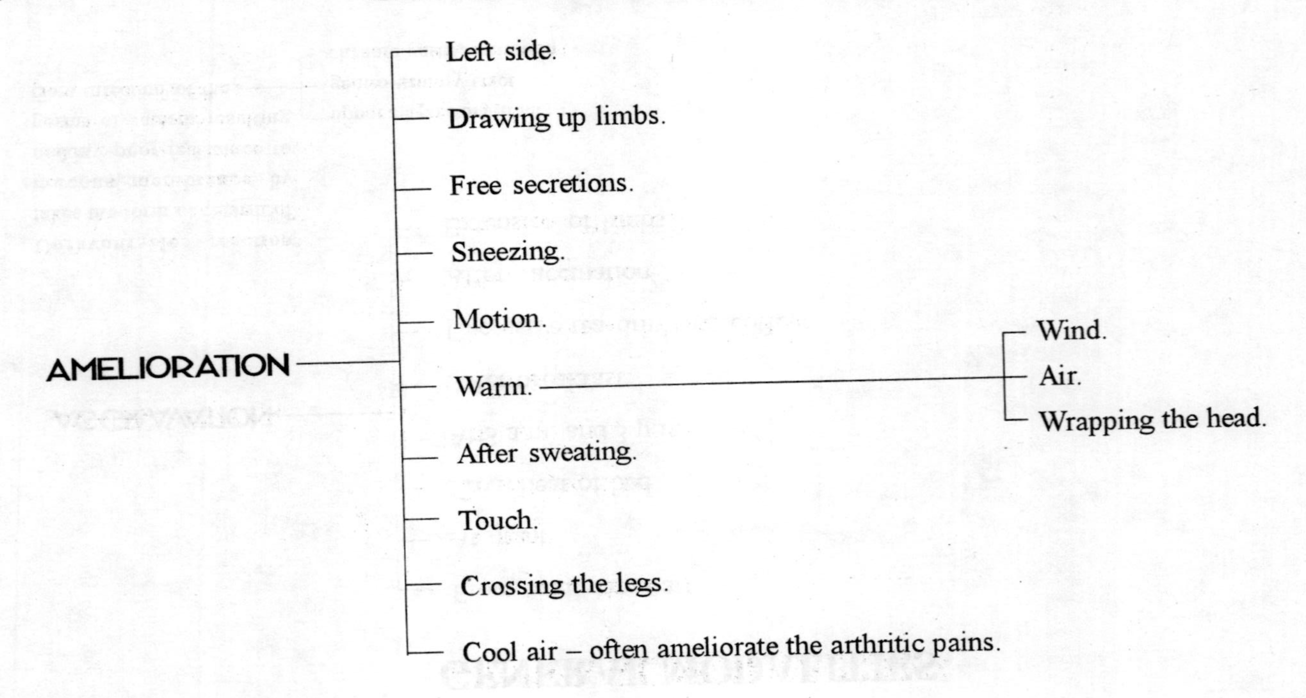

FRIEND, GURU, PHILOSOPHER

INTRODUCTION

According to Hahnemann, it is a king of anti-sycotic medicine. But it also covers psoric and syphilitic miasm in lesser degree like Tubercular diathesis.

The duration of action of even the smallest doses is nearly three weeks. It is not a safe drug in careless or ignorant hands. The diseases where the remedy is persisted in, may also become chronic. According to Kent, we will quote... "if you repeat again and again, you will have that which will remain life time. Crude drugs do not impress the vital force so lastingly but an individual who is thoroughly sensitive and properly sensitive, as sensitive as contagion, then if you undertake to prove (in potency by giving it night and morning), you will revert upon him a life-long miasm".

Usually symptomatology of Thuja is covered by *phlegmatic*[1] and *melancholic*[2] temperament. It has got tremendous power to antidote the poison of vaccination. I have seen Dr. J.N. Kanjilal, Dr. J.N. Majumdar and Dr. B.N. Chakraborty to cure many incurable diseases by a dose of Thuja occidentalis in cases with a history of repeated vaccinations as well as in those cases which were improved by indicated remedy but did not fully regain health.

---

[1] Dull and sluggish temperament.

[2] Depressed and unhappy with abnormal inhibition of mental and body activity.

Post-vaccination complications without symptomatic indication (which may be absent) or the *history of repeated vaccination* is enough, as an indication, for prescribing Thuja.[1]

Dr. R.K. Mukherjee said in his article, published in different journals, "Constitution and Temperament"; that in a deep seated constitutional dyscrasia[2] we have found excellent results from the use of *Sulphur* for a few weeks to be followed by *Thuja* for a period of few weeks and then going back to *Sulphur*.

But I have got no such experience or confirmation from my clinical practice as well as I never saw the great masters of India in general and particular to Kolkata prescribe in similar manner.

According to Tyler, remedy of 'like symptoms' is merely a vital stimulus to start a curative reaction in the patient, and required to be given only in the minimal, infrequent dose that has been established by 100 years of experience as being the most suitable for the purpose. You are using cell-poisons; and here, according to the Arndt – Schultz law, large doses may be lethal, smaller doses inhibit, while smallest doses stimulate.

---

1 **What should we search on the left arm?**

Either you get the history that first vaccination was not fully taken or a very large vaccination scar. (Dr. L.M. Khan).

2 Morbid general state, resulting from the presence of toxic matter in the blood.

FRIENDS OF THUJA OCCIDENTALIS

TRIO OF CONDYLOMATA OR FIGWARTS :

THUJA OCCIDENTALIS, STAPHYSAGRIA AND NITRICUM ACIDUM

SEQUENTIAL PRESCRIBING :

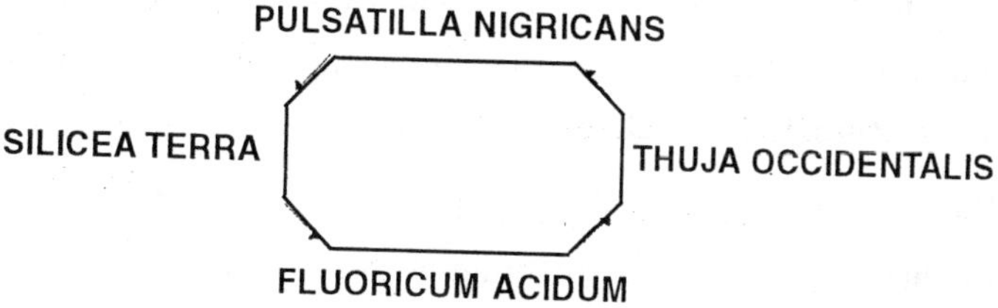

PULSATILLA NIGRICANS → THUJA OCCIDENTALIS → FLUORICUM ACIDUM → SILICEA TERRA → PULSATILLA NIGRICANS

SILICEA TERRA	THUJA OCCIDENTALIS
• More deep acting.	• Stimulates the proliforation of epithelium – its ulcers are generally superficial.
• Similar to – Many particular. – Some of the generals.	• Discharges; sweetish, offensive usually, not corrosive.
• Acts – Connective tissues. – Bones = destructive changes, suppuration. – Greater power to soften indurated tissues - its ulcers eat deeply.	• Fixed ideas – Delusions as to his persons.
• Proliferation restricted to exostosis and dnchondromata	• Modalities are more important to differenciate the both.
• Dischages; sour, putrid	
• Fixed ideas – Mania of hunting pins.	

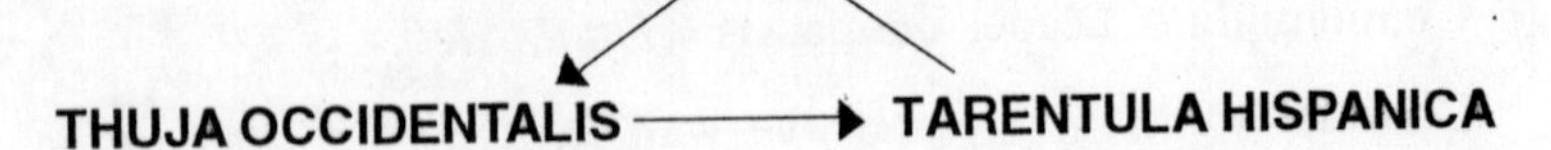

Abrotanum – Ranula.

Ammonium carbonicum – Asthma due to suppressed eczema or vaccination.

Anacardium orientale – Dissociative disorders and multiple personality.

Antimonium crudum – Plantar warts. Horny warts, sensitive to touch.

Antimonium tartaricum – Warts behind glans penis. Ill-effects of vaccination (*Maland., Vac., Vario., Kali-m., Sulph., Mez.*).

Argentum nitricum – Hurried and worried (*Med.*).

Aurum metallicum – Has a relationship with dead; dreams of them (*Zinc.*).

Baryta carbonica – Sclerosis[1] (*Con., Caust., Petr.*).

Berberis vulgaris – Severe pain at the conclusion of micturition (*Sars., Med., Equis.*).

Bryonia alba – Migraine, left sided (*Lach., Sep.*).

Calcarea carbonica – Papilloma[2] (*Thuja* especially in mouth). Relapsing otitis media; vascular tumours; relief from touching painful parts.

Carbo vegetabilis – Blackish patches/areas caused by stagnation in venules and capillaries. Pigmentary naevus (Vascular naevus-*Thuj.*).

Carcinosinum – History of severe reaction to vaccination in past or present; side effects of vaccination; imaginary pregnancy.

---

1 Term used in pathology to describe abnormal hardening or fibrosis of a tissue.

2 Benign tumor derived from epithelium.

Causticum – Warts at the junction of skin and mucous membrane; < full moon (*Cup.* – spasm).

Chamomilla – Diaper dermatitis. (*Thuj.*, *Med.*).

Cholesterinum – Hypertensive with hydrogenoid constitution.

Cinnabaris – Warts on prepuce. Horny, reddish warts.

Dulcamara – Warts fleshy, large, smooth, on the face and palmar surface of hands.

Daphne indica – Asthmatic patient with tendency for warts; bad effects of getting wet. (*Nat-s.*, *Rhus-t.*, *Rhod.*)

Equisetum hyemale – Frequènt, intolerable urging to urinate with severe pain at the close of micturition. (*Berb*, *Sars*, *Thuj.*).

Fluoricum acidum – Subinguinal blemishes (*Caust*, *Graph*, *Coli Med.*, *Nit-ac.*)

Flouricum acidum is a remedy for :–

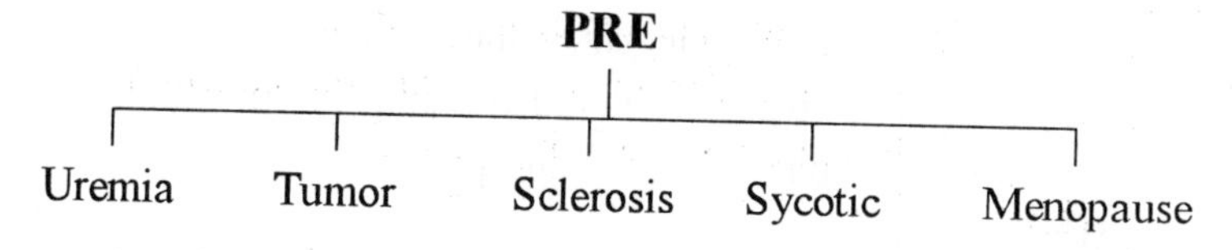

Graphites – Hypertrophy of keloid[1], cicatrices.

Hedera helix – Affection of the pancreas (*Iris-v*, *Calc.-f.*, *Phos*).

Ignatia amara – Headache as if a nail was driven out through the side of head; worse, inclining the head forward.

Kalium bromatum – Juvenile acne (*Eug.*).

Kalium chloricum – Cancerous tendency; affection at the site of vaccicinal scars.

Kreosotum – Caries in teeth (*Staph*).

Magnesium muriaticum – Warts (*Mag-s.*)

---

[1] Sharply elevated, irregularly shaped progressively enlarging scar due to excessive collagen formation in the corium during connective tissue repair.

Medorrhinum – Bad effects of repeated vaccination and intense chemotheraphy. Sudden appearance of excessive hair on limbs (*Thuj.*). Small, pointed warts.

Mercurius solubilis – Urethritis; rheumatism; condylomata of iris. Gonorrhoeal proctitis[1]. Polyp & fungus excrescence in the external meatus (*Teuc.*, *Thuj.*). Otalgia, worse from warmth of the bed.

Mercurius corrosivus – Condylomata (*Nit-ac.*)

Natrium muriaticum – Hyperglycemia as well as hypoglycemia. Sad, introverted; involvement of deepest emotional level. Leucorrhoea after chemotherapy. Hair on child's face (*Ol-j.*). Face – oily, shiny, as if greased (*Plb*, *Thuj.*).

Natrium sulphuricum – Hydrogenoid constitution. Granular lids. Green pus & terrible photophobia.

Nitricum acidum – Diarrhoea after antibiotics (*Thuj.*).

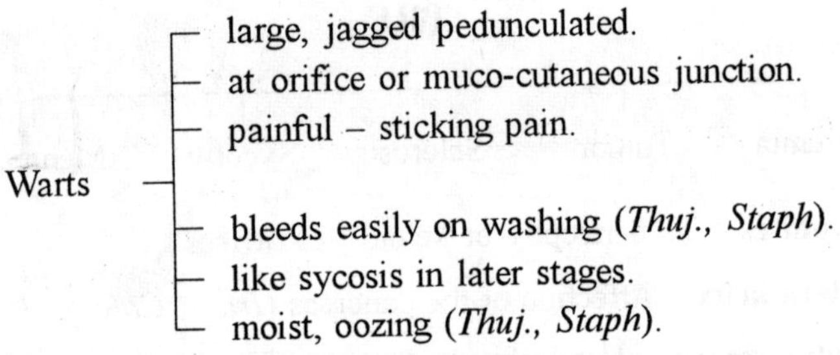

Nux vomica – Abuse of medication. Bad effects of prolonged use of corticoids (*Nat-s.*)

Opium – General sluggishnes, all sensations diminished (*Sil.*, *Thuj.*). Obstinate constipation; no desire to go to stool from inactivity or paresis of the rectum. Faeces protrude and recede (*Sil.*, *Thuj.*). Constipation from lead poisoning. Round, hard, black balls like stool (*Thuj.*, *Chel.*, *Plb.*).

---

[1] Inflammation of the rectum due to gonorrhoea.

Phosphorous – Fatty liver (*Lyc., Nat-s.*).

Platina metallicum – Coition extremely painful due to dryness of private parts.

Psorinum – Patient susceptible to glandular and skin diseases, where the indicated remedy fails.

Pulsatilla pratensis – Ozena[1], gleet[2], orchitis, prostatitis and gonorrhoea with yellowish discharge. Sterility in male. "Mild, gentle" personality and other general symptoms.

Pyrogenium – Multiple vaccinations (If sycotic – *Thuj.*; if psoric – *Sil.*)

Rauwolfia serpentina – Catarrh of mucous membrane in hypertensive patient.

Ratanhia peruviana – Pain after stool as if splincters of glass were sticking in the rectum or anus (*Thuj.*).

Sabal serrulata – Prostatic adenoma[3] (*Bar-c., Lyc.*).

Sabina – Music is intolerable; causes nervousness; goes through bone and marrow.

Sanicula aqua – Constipation with no desire until large accumulation occurs. After great straining only partially stool is expelled and then recedes (*Sil., Thuj.*). Large evacuation of small, dry grey balls; must be removed mechanically.

Sarsaparilla efficinalis – Severe, unbearable pain at the conclusion of micturition. Lack of reaction in chronic cases. Affections of right kidney (affection of left kidney – *Berb-v.*).

Scarlatinum – After vaccination; involvement of the kidneys, and rheumatism.

Sepia officinalis – Dyspepsia of tea and tobacco drinkers. Painful warts, hirsutism[4], dyspepsia, ptosis.

---

[1] Atrophic rhinitis marked by thick mucopurulent discharge, and fetor.

[2] Mucus discharge from the urethra in chronic gonorrhoea.

[3] Benign enlargement of the prostate gland.

[4] Abnormal hairiness, especially in women.

Personality profile : Females with narrow hips and masculine appearance; moustachoid ladies.

Males rarely requires shaving and have typical feminine pelvis.

Silicea terra – Small pox when suppuration started. Ill effects of vaccination; effects of impure vaccination. Long lasting diarrhoea after vaccination. BCG vaccination causes intolerance; after vaccination, tonsillar hypertrophy. Brittle nails (Cylinder, brittle & crumbling nails – *Thuj.*).

Constipation — Stool partly expelled & then recedes.
Always before & during menses.
Due to inactivity of the rectum with great straining.

Staphysagria – Hypertrophy of the prostate (*Sel.*, *Lyc.*, *Thuj.*)

Figwart —
- after abuse of mercury (*Nit-ac.*, *Sabin.*, *Thuj.*)
- pedunculated, dry;
- like cauliflower.

Sulphur – In gonorrhoea, when other remedies fail (*Med.*). To bring back the suppressed discharges which was ameliorated (*Med.*, *Puls.* – warts in hot blooded persons; *Thuj.* – useful in warts in chilly patient).

Movement in abdomen as of a child (*Croc.*, *Thuj.*).

Cupped teeth in children. Crumbled teeth; yellow; decay easily.

Syphilinum – Fissures in the rectum and anus (*Thuj.*)

Prolapse of rectum; obstinate cases with history of syphilis.

Teucrium marum verum – Polypus at the neck of uterus (*Nit-ac.*)

Thlapsi bursa pastoris – In renal lithiasis[1].

Theridion curassavicum – Sensitive to least noise. Vertigo on closing eyes (*Lach.*, *Thuj.*). Chronic nasal catarrh with thick,

[1] Condition marked by formation of calculi and concretions in the kidneys.

yellow, greenish, offensive discharge (*Puls.*, *Thuj.*).

Variolinum – Pitting of skin after small pox.

THUJA AS A GURU

Aurum muriaticum natronatum – Induration, hypertrophy of female genitalia (*Aurum-m. k.*).

Berberis vulgaris – Liver, kidney, skin.

Causticum – In cystic tumours.

Chimaphila umbellata – Hypertrophy, induration, chronic infection with flaky urine.

Dulcamara – Acute complaints of tonsils with hypertrophy due to bad effects of vaccination.

Formica rufa – Coli bacillus infection in urine.

Hydrastis canadensis – Portal congestion.

Iodium – Hard glandular growth; cancerous development, etc.

Kalium bichromicum – Renal colic with albuminuria, oliguria[1], nephritis with pain in urethra during and after micturition.

Lachesis mutus – Neuro– endocrine disorders of puberty; liver complaint; left ovary; varicosities; fibroma.

Medorrhinum – Thuja does not complete the cure – chronic rheumatism, sycotic discharges after acute phase. Personal history of urethritis, etc.

Natrium muriaticum – Hypotrophy in infants. Late learning to talk.

Natrium sulphuricum – Sycotic syndromes. Deep-seated sycotic constitutional deficiency where the sycotic condition is associated with hydrogenoid. Neuralgia, rheumatism, diarrhoea.

---

[1] Diminished urine secretion in relation to fluid intake.

Nitricum acidum – Vesical polypus (*Calc.*).

Petroselinum sativum – Cystitis, calculi.

Rhus toxicodendron – Lumbo-sacral pain; worse, wet rainy weather.

Hydrogenoid constitution; better, heat and continued motion (*Dulc.*)

Sabal serrulata – Adenoma of prostrate (*Bar-c.*).

Sabina – Sycotic skin excresences with gonorrheal rheumatism. Lumbo-sacral pain associated with haemorrhages in female due to polypus & with dysmenorrhoea.

Sarsaparilla officinalis – Intolerable pain at the conclusion of micturition.

Selenium metallicum – Abuse of tea; genito-urinary disorder; sub-orbital neuralgia.

Sepia officinalis – Chronic urinary infection (*Arg-n.*, *Ars.*, *Canth.*, *Equis-h.*, *Merc-c.*, *Nit-ac.*).

Silicea terra – Nervous disorder. For bad effects of vaccination. Suppuration; weakness, emaciation; poor immunity. Marfan's disease[1].

Staphysagria – Burning in urethra; relieved by urination; cystitis, prostatic involvement, etc.

Tuberculinum – Useful remedy for deep action in personal or family history of Koch's.

---

[1] **Marfan's disease : Hereditary syntrome of abnormal length of the extremities especially of finger & toes with subluxation of the lens, cardio-vascular abnormalities and other disorders.** *(Ref : Dorland's Medical Dictionary).*

WHEN THUJA FAILS

Alumina – Constipation in women with very sedentary habits. Loose, party stool passed with difficulty; great straining. History of prolonged gonorrhoea with palliative medicine like *Puls.*

Antimonium tartaricum – Bad effects of vaccination when *Thuj.* fails and *Sil.* is not indicated.

Apis mellifica – Intermittent fever and symptoms related to prostate gland.

Arsenicum album – Filarial fever with painful swelling of lower extremities especially right knee.

Baryta carbonica – Enlarged tonsil with history of vaccination when *Sil.* fails.

Calcarea calcinata – In warts cases when *Thuj.* and *Caust.* fails.

Calcarea phosphorica – Enlarged tonsils; desires fatty meat, salt; blackish, tall person.

Carcinosinum – When *Thuj.* seems apparently to be prescribed accurately but proves worthless. Case perceiving shows combination of many personality profiles/portrait of disease.

Castoreum – Warts, when *Nat-s.* and *Thuj.* fails.

Causticum – In cases of crops of warts found around the genitals.

Chimaphila umbellata – Chronic infection in the urinary tract, enlarged prostate; induration.

Lachesis mutus – Removal of injected poisons as well as other animal poisoning like rat bite, snake bite, etc. and their post effects.

Lapis albus – In goitre.

Mercurius solubilis – Removal of injected poisons, animal poisons, etc. Small pox when suppuration started.

Natrium sulphuricum – Asthma.

Niticum acidum – Gleet with darting pain and condylomata; anal fissure.

Phosphoricum acidum – Dejected mood with gonorrhoea; prostration, weakness, etc.

Psorinum – Case of unilateral arrest of development; poor development of left breast.

Sabina – Warty, fleshy excrescences in left side of mouth. Condylomata and sycotic affections.

Sepia officinalis – Small valvety warts on penis especially around the prepuce.

Silicea terra – Straight and brittle nails (Hard nails – *Thuj.*). Complaints due to suppressed abscess at the rectum, especially fistula. Skin disease; chilly; sensitive; shy. Tendency to catch cold easily.

Staphysagria – Figwarts and condylomata due to abuse of mercury especially when *Thuj.* fails.

Stellaria media – Wonderful remedy when not only *Thuj.*; *Merc.*, *Aur.* fail.

Sulphur – Deep seated constitutional deficiency. Post vaccination complications. *Thuj.* or *Maland.* are not enough for removal of injected poison or animal or other poisons. Involuntary seminal discharge, relaxed testicles hanging down with sweating around the scrotum and between the scrotum and thighs.

Syphilinum – Retarded growth.

Tuberculinum bovinum kent – Tubercular background or personal history of Kochs. Deep constitutional deficiency with tubercular diathesis when even *Merc-s.* and *Sulph.* fail.

Variolinum – Eczema after vaccination.

BIBLIOGRAPHY

- 'Organon – The Art of Healing' : Samuel Hahnemann. (Translated by R.E. Dudgeon); 6th edition; Pratap Medical Publishers, 1994.
- Allen, H.C., Keynotes and Characteristics with Comparisons of some of the Leading Remedies of the Materia Medica; 5th Indian edition; Economic Homoeo Publishers.
- Boger C.M., a synoptic Key of Materia Medica, sixth edition, Salzen & Co., Calcutta.
- Boeninghausen C.M. & Boger C.M., Boeninghausen's Characteristics & Repertory, Second edition, Roy & Co., Bombay, 1952.
- Boger, C.M., Study of Materia Medica and Case Taking; B.Jain Publishers, New Delhi, 1992.
- Borland, D.M., Homoeopathy in Theory & Practice, Roy & Co., Bombay.
- Gallavardin J.P., Psychisme et Homoeopathie 1960. (German translation : Horst Barthel, 1986)
- Boericke, O.E., Pocket Manual of Homoeopathic Materia Medica, sixth edition, Boericke & Runyon, New York, 1916.
- Allen T.F., The Encyclopedia of pure Materia Medica, Boericke & Tafel, New York, Philadelphia, 1874-1879.

- Clarke, J.H., A Dictionary of Practical Materia Medica, The Homoeopathic Publishing Co., London, 1947.
- Choudhary, N.M., A Study on Materia Medica, B.Jain Publishers, 1995.
- Gentry, W.D., The Concordance Repertory, Chatterton & Co., New York, 1890.
- Dewey, W.A., Essentials of Homoeopathic Materia Medica, k. edition, 1908.
- Guernsey, H.N., Keynotes to Materia Medica, Boericke, Philadelphia, 1887.
- Hering C., The Guiding Symptoms of our Materia Medica, 1870-1891.
- Nash, E.B., Leaders in Homoeopathic Therapeutics, Boericke & Tafel, Philadelphia, 1898.
- Tyler, M.L., Homoeopathic Drug Pictures, Boericke & Tafel, London, 1952.
- Lippe, A.von, Dr. Lippe's Charakteristische symptome, hrsg., durch T.L. Bradford, Hang verlag, Heidelberg, 1967.
- Hughes, R. & Dake, J.P., A Cyclopedia of Drug Pathogenesy, 1886.
- Hughes, R. & Dake, The knowledge of Physicians, 1884, Reprinted by B.Jain Publishers, New Delhi.
- Kent, J.T., Lectures on Homoeopathic Philosophy, B.Jain Publishers, New Delhi.
- Dhawale, M.L., Principles & Practice of Homoeopathy, 1967.
- Fritj of Capra : The Turning Point.
- Gypser, K.H., Kent's Minor Writings on Homoeopathy, B.Jain Publishers, New Delhi, India.
- Whitmond, Edward C., Psyche and Substance.

- Clarke, A dictionary of Practical Materia Medica.
- Allen, H.C., Keynotes with nosodes.
- Allen, T.F.
- Boericke.
- Boger.
- Clarke, J.
- Dunham, C., Homoeopathy. The Science of Therapeutics.
- Farrington, E.A., Comparative Materia Medica & Clinical Materia Medica.
- Hughes, R., Pharmacodynamics.
- Kent, J.T.
- Neat by & Stoneham, Manual.
- Roberts, H.A., Rheumatic remedies.
- Tyler, M.L., Hahnemann conception of chronic diseases.
- Weir, Sir, John, Homoeopathy – An explanation of its principles.

EARLY DEVELOPMENT OF THUJA PROVING

1 HAHNEMANN (in Reine Arzmittelheire, Vol. V of original, Vol.II of translation).

Contains
- Self – 334 symptoms.
- 10 Fellow provers – 300 symptoms.
  ↓
  (Franz, Gross, Fr. Hahnemann, Hartmann, Haynel, Hempel, Langhammer, Teuthorn, Wagner, Wislicenus).

2 BOHM
- Nov. 12th, 1884 (1st time).
- After two & half months (2nd time proving).

3 FROHLICH; six separate provings
- Dec. 20th, 1844.
- Jan. 2nd, 1845.
- Jan. 22nd, 1845.
- April 4th, 1845.
- April 22nd, 1845.
- May 21st, 1845.

4 CAROLINE P.
- Nov. 12th, 1844 (self).
- Dec. 12th, 1844 (2 provers).

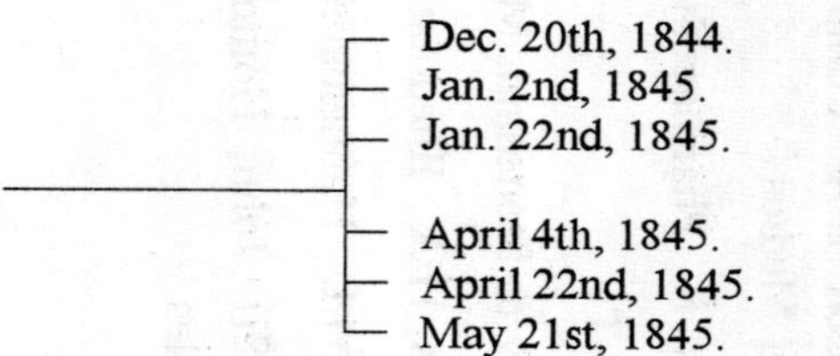

No.	Prover	Dates
5	WILLIAM HUBER of Linz (in different doses; from grain doses to 60th dilution)	12th Sept., 1844. 30th Sept., 1844. Jan. 16th, 1845.
6	W. HUBER (Brother of William Huber; Surgeon of Kleinzell)	Self, 2 females (one his wife), 3 his children.
	In different ages, sex and in different doses, he proved the medicine.	April 19th, 1845. June 18th, 1845. 18th May, 1845. 14th Sept., 1845. 3rd May to 7th Dec., 1845.
7	F. LACKNER, Student of Medicine	Oct, 10th, 1844 – Dec., 1844. Jan. 8th – Feb. 8th.
8	J. LANDESMANN (Physician)	Sept. – Dec., 1844. Feb. 1845.
9	Dr. and Prof. LIEDBECK (42 yrs. old)	Sept., 1844.
10	Dr. MASCHAUER	Sept. 21st – Nov. 8th, 1844. Dec. 5th – Jan. 2nd, 1845.

No.	Prover	Dates
11	Dr. MAYRHOFER (Self & his wife)	Sept./Nov./Dec., 1844.
12	MARIA ANNA	June 17th, 1845.
13	Dr. REISINGER	Nov. 5th, 1844. March 1st, 1845. 3rd time.
14	Dr. STERZ	Oct. 13th, 1844. Dec., 1844.
15	WACHTEL (Proved in dilution only)	Dec. 10th, 1844. Jan. 8th, 1845.
16	WATZKE	Nov. 1844. Dec. 19th, 1844. Jan. 1845. Feb. 5th, 1845. Feb. 25th, 1845.
17	Dr. WURHB (4 with mother tincture, 1 with dilution)	Sept. 1844, Dec. 1844.

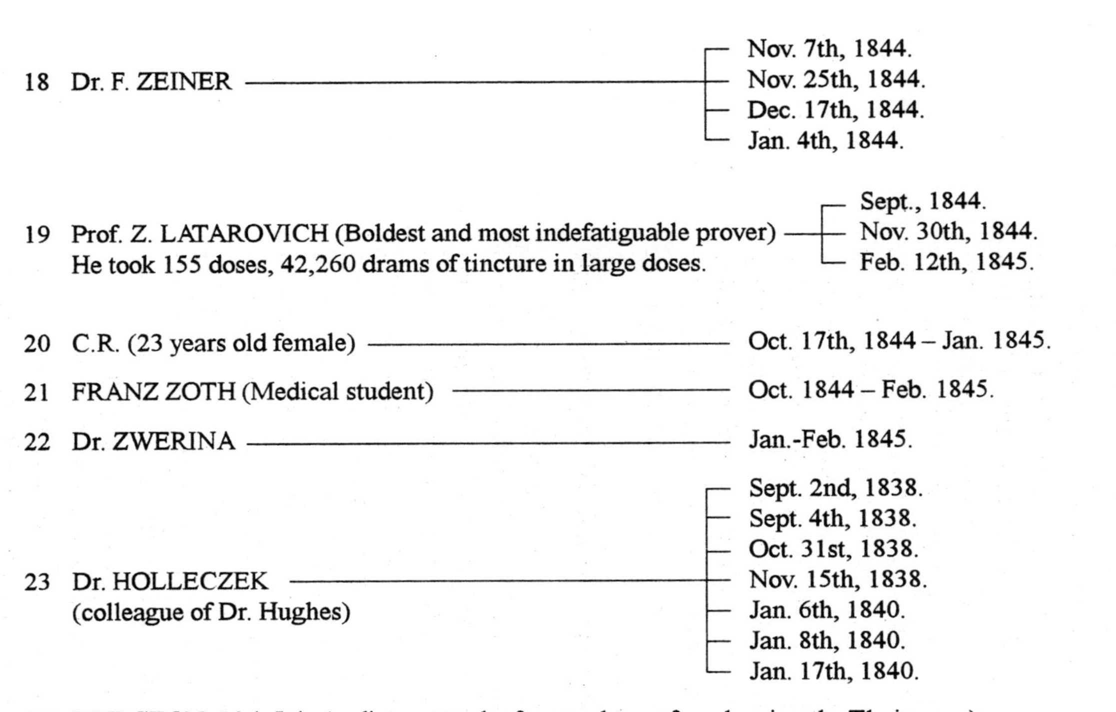

No.	Prover	Dates
18	Dr. F. ZEINER	Nov. 7th, 1844. Nov. 25th, 1844. Dec. 17th, 1844. Jan. 4th, 1844.
19	Prof. Z. LATAROVICH (Boldest and most indefatiguable prover) He took 155 doses, 42,260 drams of tincture in large doses.	Sept., 1844. Nov. 30th, 1844. Feb. 12th, 1845.
20	C.R. (23 years old female)	Oct. 17th, 1844 – Jan. 1845.
21	FRANZ ZOTH (Medical student)	Oct. 1844 – Feb. 1845.
22	Dr. ZWERINA	Jan.-Feb. 1845.
23	Dr. HOLLECZEK (colleague of Dr. Hughes)	Sept. 2nd, 1838. Sept. 4th, 1838. Oct. 31st, 1838. Nov. 15th, 1838. Jan. 6th, 1840. Jan. 8th, 1840. Jan. 17th, 1840.
24	DUDGEON, 10th July (ordinary attack of gonorrhoea after chewing the Thuja cone)	

SUBSCRIPTION COUPON

Yes, I would like to renew/subscribe to

The Homoeopathic Heritage

Price

Annual	Life Members (10 years)
Rs. 200 (India, Nepal, Bhutan)	Rs. 1500 (India, Nepal, Bhutan)
US$ 15 (Bangladesh)	US$ 100 (Bangladesh)
US$ 20 (Pakistan)	US$ 150 (Pakistan)
US$ 25 (Rest of the World)	US$ 200 (Rest of the World)

MODE OF PAYMENT

For India, Nepal & Bhutan by M.O., Bank Draft or Cheque payable at Delhi, New Delhi in favour of **B. Jain Publishers (P) Ltd.,** 1921/10, Chuna Mandi, Paharganj, Post Box 5775, New Delhi-55, India.

For Overseas by International Money Order or Bank Draft in favour of **B. Jain Publishers Overseas,** 1920, Street No. 10, Chuna Mandi, Paharganj, Post Box 5775, New Delhi-55, India.

You can pay through credit card also.

WRITE IN CAPITALS

Name..

Complete Mailing Address..............................

....

....

....Pin ....

Renewal ☐

(Old Subs. No........)

New ☐

Ph. (Res.) .... Ph.(Off.)..

E-mail ....

I am remitting Rs./US$ .... by M.O./ Bank draft/cheque.

Please charge it to my (✓) Visa/Master/American Express Card No.

☐☐☐☐☐☐☐☐☐☐☐☐☐☐☐☐ VISA MasterCard

Card Expiry ☐☐ ☐☐
MM YY

Date.................... Signature